T0147161

FROM CFS WITH LOVE

Techniques to relieve and release symptoms of Chronic Fatigue Syndrome, Fibromyalgia and Chemical Sensitivities

KARYL M SANCHEZ

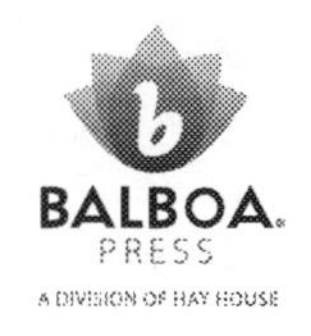

Balboa Press books may be ordered through booksellers or by contacting:

Balboa Press
A Division of Hay House
1663 Liberty Drive
Bloomington, IN 47403
www.balboapress.com
1 (877) 407-4847

Print information available on the last page.

ISBN: 978-1-5043-5619-0 (sc)
ISBN: 978-1-5043-5621-3 (hc)
ISBN: 978-1-5043-5620-6 (e)

Library of Congress Control Number: 2016906356

Balboa Press rev. date: 07/11/2016

DEDICATION

I dedicate this book to all sufferers of Chronic Fatigue Syndrome, Fibromyalgia and Chemical Sensitivities. There have been many names given to this syndrome such as Yuppy Flu, Myalgic Encephalitis and others, however, the "dis-ease" is the same. (not being at ease).

CHANGE COMES WITH COURAGE
AND COURAGE COMES WITH CHANGE

Courage comes after you have experienced Pride, Anger, Desire, Fear, Grief, Apathy, Guilt, Shame. (a quote from David R. Hawkins, M.D., Ph.D. in his book Power vs Force).

With the determination and aspiration to experience the emotional spiral going up instead of down, we are encouraged to encounter more healing, more positive and lighter filled emotions, such as neutrality, willingness, acceptance, reason, love, joy, peace, and enlightenment when dealing with healing from Chronic Fatigue Syndrome.

Contribute and make a commitment to heal yourself. As you heal yourself you will encourage others revealing that healing from CFS is possible.

CONTENTS

ABOUT THE AUTHOR

I write this book not because Chronic Fatigue Syndrome is considered an untreatable medical condition, but because I believe in our bodies, instinctive ability to heal themselves, and by using practical, intuitive and complimentary medicines to do so, as well as taking 100 percent responsibility for our own healing.

I was diagnosed with Chronic Fatigue Syndrome and Fibromyalgia. The doctors words were "go to sleep," and that he could do nothing for me. I asked "how long for?" He looked at me, pondered and said, "maybe two years," I found that outrageous but had no strength to argue, and so found myself with no strength to do much at all for the first two to three years, I could not even pick up a book to research Chronic Fatigue Syndrome. My family had no idea and I was unable to communicate with them the extent of what I was feeling.

Through determination and a strong desire to heal, I am here today giving you all I can on this subject and hope to inspire you into healing.

With Love

Karyl

FOREWORD

I'm thrilled and excited that Karyl has decided to share her experiences of recovering from Chronic Fatigue Syndrome (CFS) with the world! Having suffered in the past from CFS myself and subsequently fully recovered, I know how difficult the condition is to deal with in day to day life. But Karyl gives people the hope and support to take a healing journey, because she can really relate to people with the condition. I first came into contact with Karyl when she took my CFS and Fibromyalgia healing course, the "Gupta Programme", where she experienced a significant increase in energy, followed by changes in other symptoms of CFS. Combined with other therapies, her body started feeling strong and staying strong, after many years of experiencing CFS. So she is brilliantly placed to help others.

This book is unique in the sense that it not only gives the reader insights of the illness through the author's experience, but as a practitioner of Kinesiology and Remedial Massage, running a Naturopathic clinic and having contact with many people with debilitating chronic illness, she developed exercises to support the process of healing. The book consists of 4 main techniques she has used to achieve her results, and I really encourage you to try them all and see what works for you. Karyl has put together various discussions and suggestions of therapies and techniques, to help the reader broaden their understanding of what works.

We all deserve the gift of a healthy body free from CFS, it is our birth right. So I encourage you to really believe in what Karyl offers, and to keep the faith that healing will come, even through your darkest hours. So onwards and upwards Brave Warrior! We all believe in you and your ability to be healthy and happy!

With Love
Ashok Gupta
Director of the Gupta Programme
www.guptaprogramme.com

INTRODUCTION

My journey with Chronic Fatigue Syndrome (CFS) and Fibromyalgia has spanned 11 years. At the time of my diagnosis, the medical advice I was given and the subsequent treatment options were ineffective in treating my symptoms. This set me on a path of gathering information, self-discovery and healing. The culmination of which is set forth in the pages of this book.

Chronic fatigue syndrome (CFS) and Fibromyalgia are medical conditions that are often difficult to diagnose and treat from a western medical approach. The information provided in this book should be considered as a guide only and does not replace the advice of qualified medical practitioners. I do encourage you to discuss any changes you choose to make with your health care practitioner.

What in fact is it about CFS and Fibromyalgia that makes it so intense?

It seems to frighten us. Why?

Perhaps it's the length of time we are sick, the many symptoms, the poor prognosis, there isn't a peak and low curve of sickness like other illnesses, such as infections or inflammations for example. The period of feeling unwell goes on and on, giving it an unnatural characteristic.

Having any chronic illness or condition changes how you experience your world. My life with CFS and Fibromyalgia had a profound effect on my development as a person, making me more "sensitive" and changing me in ways I could not have envisaged. This sensitivity I speak of encompasses not only the physical body. I became more emotionally, spiritually and even psychically sensitive. The latter was perhaps the biggest change for me to deal with.

It became very clear to me that I needed to stop and re-assess my whole life. Through this process, I learnt the importance of viewing this experience with love and as a gift.

One of the tools in the aid of changing perspective is, love. Love is felt effortlessly, you can show love or experience love suddenly and without a thought process. So what I am trying to explain here is perhaps, contemplate an effortless process of belief in the release of the very real and unquestionable symptoms you experience, see these leave your everyday life by showing love to the experience of CFS and leaving fear behind.

I found the first step towards recovery is changing your perception of CFS. See the illness with softness and love, relax and hold a strong belief that these symptoms will be released from your everyday experience.

The need, the imperative necessity of change is undoubtable and clear, we need to detox (1), learn and develop techniques to calm the central nervous system (2) and discover ways to take care of our bodies so we can cope with the environmental stimuli (3).

Tiny, little insignificant twinkles of miracles is how I would now describe the changes I began to experience when the symptoms started to change. They certainly were not overnight but week by week and month by month I could notice the changes. Something like this:

Breath improved.

Gut function improved, bloating, constipation, nausea the cramped stomach muscles.

The lymphatic system changed, there was a tightening of the skin around the arm pits, the stomach, the neck, even the ankles and wrists.

The body's response to chemicals improved.

The muscle pain started to disappear sometimes it comes and goes for a short time, not like the everyday experience.

The sore throat went away and the glands were not raw red and inflamed.

The headaches finally disappeared.

The overactive brain and the sleep patterns of crashing and then waking up and not being able to go back to sleep has changed.

The strength returned, when you can throw something across the room you know you are getting better.

The humour returned, it's nice to be silly again and find joy in your day.

Finally reading again without exhausting your eyes and actually enjoying it.

Getting your memory back, short term and the long term.

Being able to go dancing, even have a cocktail or two again.

One of the symptoms I have experienced has not changed the emotional sensitivity. HSP is the term used to describe it, highly sensitive people, which is believed, 20% of the population experiences. Some children are born like this and some adults develop it, you will find more on this subject in the sensitivities chapter.

As you begin to notice the symptoms subsiding your power will increase and your energy will show up.

In this book I discuss the 4 techniques that worked for me and I hope it will work for you. They are; Colonics, detox diet, herbs and The Amygdala Retraining Program.

I found that giving some background explanation on some of the systems affected by CFS such as the immune system, the lymphatic system, the endocrine system, for example, may give you more insight and understanding on the techniques and tools I put forward to help the body in maintenance and support.

I discuss some tools I gathered during my research and experience working as a Kinesiologist and Remedial Massage practitioner together with the many therapies that I have come across in the process of healing.

I put forward my theory of CFS and note some theories that have been put forward by others.

I found a need for some sort of structure or instrument to assist in aiding the central nervous system as well as the huge array of symptoms faced by the CFS sufferer hence the reason I have scattered exercises within this book, to use as tools for support.

I had to assess what was working for me and what was not.

It is necessary for each person to do that, to look at themselves and go within to find answers for recovery. It is definitely a personal journey.

Even though I give you many exercises and tools to make life easier with your CFS symptoms at the end of the day it is up to you, where you find the strength to develop faith in healing.

THANK YOU

There are some very individual, courageous and passionate people pioneering exploring and developing theories on CFS, like Dr Liz Lipski (USA) with her work on the gut function and Dr Sarah Myhill (London) with her theory on the mitochondria. As they share their knowledge and inspiration in the medical field it makes CFS sufferer's world a better place, more united giving us long needed hope. I make reference to their work because it is so profoundly relevant to CFS sufferers. There are so many more like, Dr Mercola (USA), Ashok Gupta (London), Donna Gates with Colon health, Dr Ian Rafter, (Sydney), even Dr Oz has some great info out there, I could make this list quite long, and deservingly so.

In the whole population of the world only a few stand out through their work as "Love builders" also referred to as "light workers." One is Louise Hay, her work on "Love the life you live," how you can love yourself more and "heal your body," is not only pioneering work on the subject of self help but simple, inspiring and invaluable.

"Change the way we perceive other people."

Dr Hew Len Ihaleakala explains that it is important to look at our own world first, if we are willing to do that, our impact on the whole Cosmos will be enormous.

Dr Hew Len felt his job was to help himself by letting go of how he perceived handicapped children. He changed his perception of handicapped children (quite like how he changed the way he perceived the mentally criminally insane at the Hawaii State Hospital in the late 80's) and with this shift of mindset "the patients" changed.

Dr Hew Len went on to stress that most people think they are here to help other people and bring peace to the world, but we are only here to bring peace to ourselves, because by bringing peace to ourselves, we bring peace to the world (and not the other way round).

Dr Hew Len says that the only thing that works is, if we look within ourselves and clear up our own imperfections. He points out that, as he does this, he notices that people get well and are able to start taking responsibility for themselves." (this extract above is from Dr Hew Len Ihaleakala's website)

Dr Hew Len's work was the inspiration for calling my book "From CFS with Love". I felt that CFS was no longer a curse but a blessing. When my attitude and outlook changed my ability to look for answers became much easier.

I am forever grateful to Dr Ian Rafter, Jon Gamble, Eli Shammon, and Dan McDonald for their expertise and attention in the process of my healing.

I also thank my family and friends who have helped me with editing and for being the wonderful people in my life.

Chapter 1

SYMPTOMS

The symptoms for Chronic Fatigue Syndrome, as you can imagine, have been debated and redefined in the last 20 years, noting the complexity of this illness.

Some people, in their considered opinion, feel that it is under classified and "Syndrome" does not allow the classification to fully describe the severity of the illness.

Personally I would recommend not get too emotionally involved in criteria and concentrate on healing.

So I leave you with the information of what Chronic Fatigue Syndrome or Fibromyalgia is and clarify what it is not.

It is not, feeling tired.

It is not, a lower back pain or neck pain.

It is not, headaches.

Or digestion problems.

Or sleep inconsistencies.

It is not about one or two of these symptoms. It is a combination and a certain length of time suffering these symptoms and much more.

It has nothing to do with feeling tired, it is fairer to say that it is like having a bad flu that does not go away for years. The tests by doctors, which come back negative; the frustrated frowns by doctors investigating your condition and the fear that you're symptoms are not believed is very hard to bare, that's why CFS is such a strange and baffling affliction.

The illness was named Chronic Fatigue Syndrome because it reflects the most common symptom — long-term, persistent fatigue. (Today, Chronic Fatigue Syndrome also is known as Myalgic Encephalomyelitis, Post viral Fatigue Syndrome, Chronic Fatigue and Immune Dysfunction Syndrome).

What are the symptoms and signs of Chronic Fatigue Syndrome?

The symptoms and signs of Chronic Fatigue Syndrome are a few but specific and consistent.

You must have severe chronic fatigue for six months or longer with other known medical conditions excluded by clinical diagnosis.

Plus the following symptoms that either occurred at the same time or after the severe chronic fatigue.

The symptoms are substantial impairment in short-term memory or concentration, sore throat, tender lymph nodes, muscle pain, multi-joint pain without swelling or redness, headaches of a new type, pattern or severity, non-refreshing sleep, and post-exertion malaise lasting more than 24 hours (be in pain after exercise or physical activity lasting more than 24 hours).

You may often have additional symptoms such as double vision, mild fevers, earaches, diarrhea, and many other symptoms, but they do not fit into the criteria that are considered to be part of the definition of CFS.

I would suggest you research the Canadian governments website, the UK definitions and also the Australian health governments description of Chronic Fatigue Syndrome. What I have noted is that they are different but have common factors. To be honest nothing really prepares you for this illness but as you research the many entangled symptoms you will start to understand how you are feeling.

The Australian government site has described a few little extra symptoms, I found interesting for example; People with CFS may feel dizzy when they stand up quickly.

They may notice that they are sensitive to some foods, smells (such as paint thinners and other chemicals), bright lights, cigarette smoke, and they may not be able to drink alcohol.

Some people with CFS find that they become unwell with infections such as colds, common viruses or flu more often than they did before they developed CFS and that it can take a long time before they feel well again.

DIAGNOSIS

There is no test which can diagnose CFS.

No specific change in the body has been found apart from some very small changes in the way that the brain works - which can only be found by very sophisticated and expensive scans.

There are many other illnesses which cause feelings of fatigue, such as some viral infections, low levels of thyroid hormone, depression, sleep apnea (obstruction of breathing while asleep), kidney disease, severe anemia, cancer, eating disorders, alcohol or other drug abuse induced symptoms, and extreme obesity.

These will need to be ruled out before a diagnosis of prolonged or chronic fatigue can be made.

Tests such as tests of ability to concentrate, think and remember could be done.

It might be recognised that the person is unwell and has severe fatigue well before 6 months has passed. This may be later recognised to be CFS, but not before 6 months has passed, the illness might be called 'prolonged fatigue' or 'chronic fatigue'.

Please note: there are variations in certain descriptions of symptoms but generally they are quite similar.

It's useful at the beginning when a person is diagnoses to understand the symptoms and the necessity to broaden the awareness of symptoms to simply understand what is happening to them.

It is so important to keep in mind that each individual has their own genetical weaknesses and characteristics, their own genetic make-up, and therefore symptoms do vary. One CFS patient may have different symptoms from another person with the same diagnosis. I have met people with CFS in different stages of the illness and some who have worked on themselves and others who have not done much at all but to take medication for depression and give up, we are all different and in my view we need to be compassionate with ourselves, be empathetic stay focussed on healing and getting better no matter how bad the symptoms are or how long they go for.

Below is Dr Sarah Myhill's list of symptoms. You can find her book on her website. "Diagnosis and Treatment of Chronic Fatigue Syndrome - It's mitochondria, not hypochondria" Published by Sarah Myhill Limited Website: www.drmyhill.co.uk

Symptoms of CFS

(Dr Myhill) "My current understanding of CFS is that it is a symptom of mitochondrial malfunction. In Part II of this book I will explain the role of mitochondria, the biochemical processes inside each cell involved in producing energy, and I will show how many of the symptoms of CFS can be explained by mitochondrial dysfunction. Then the references I make here to mitochondria, ATP, ADP, cell-free DNA etc. will become much clearer. First, however, let us look at the clinical picture of the illness.

The two key symptoms in patients with CFS which I believe reflect the mitochondrial dysfunction are:

Very poor stamina (mental and physical) – i.e. you can do things, but only for about 5 seconds before tiring. This is due to slow recycling of ATP (see p.9).

Delayed fatigue (mental and physical) – i.e. symptoms persist for 24 - 96 hours if you over-do things. This is because when mitochondria are stressed, all the energy molecules (ATP, ADP and AMP) are drained out and cells have to wait 1-4 days for new energy molecules to be made via the pentose phosphate shunt.

These two symptoms are central to the diagnosis of CFS. The mental fatigue manifests as poor short term memory, inability to follow a line of argument, difficulty reading or watching TV, poor problem solving ability, difficulty dealing with more than one thing at a time – what I call foggy brain. As one of my patients put it: "Nothing right in my left brain, nothing left in my right brain!"

In additions to the above, there are common symptoms present in many cases. These symptoms are worsened when the patient overdoes things:

Malaise (i.e. a feeling of illness) – this is caused by damage to tissues when the sufferer overdoes things. In tests this is reflected by a high level of cell-free DNA, which is a measure of tissue damage (cf. p. 17). See also INFLAMMATION.

Muscle pain - ditto – also caused by poor antioxidant status, early switch into anaerobic metabolism, or magnesium deficiency. See PAIN, FIBROMYALGIA, ALLERGIC MUSCLES, STIFF MUSCLES.

Muscle weakness (including the muscles in the eyes giving episodic, variable, blurring of vision).

Sleep disturbance (whereby the "biological clock" is moved on 1-6 hours and CFSs drop off to sleep late and wake late). CFS sufferers are natural owls.

Tendency to get recurrent infections – see VIRAL INFECTIONS – HOW TO AVOID a general hypersensitivity to noise, light, touch, pain, smells etc drug and alcohol intolerance – a small drink gives a big hangover. Indeed intolerance of many drugs is common especially to antidepressants, beta blockers, statins and blood pressure medication. This may reflect poor detoxification pathway with stressing of the P450 enzymes and an out-pouring of free radicals. However many of these substances inhibit mitochondria directly or worsen the already struggling low cardiac output. See DETOXIFICATION feeling of "not being with it" poor temperature control gut symptoms: ALLERGY, HYPOGLYCEMIA, GUT DYSBIOSIS, HYPOCHLORYDRIA, YEAST PROBLEMS, MALABSORPTION, POOR PANCREATIC FUNCTION, HYDROGEN SULPHIDE, FERMENTATION IN THE GUT.

Headache.

Mood swings – see BRAIN IN CFS – EDGE EFFECT.

Joint pain – see NUTRITIONAL TREATMENT OF ARTHRITIS, OSTEOPOROSIS.

There are usually few physical signs. Sometimes there are tender trigger points in muscles and tendons, sometimes signs of inflammation such as swollen tender lymph nodes in the neck or low-grade fever. However, often there are no obvious abnormalities on physical examination – indeed, the patient may look reasonably well.

Depression is not part of CFS but can arise in any patient who has been chronically ill with "no light at the end of the tunnel." The main cause of depression in CFS patients results from bad treatment by their physicians. It disturbs me that so many physicians feel able to send their patients away with no coherent sensible management plan or glimmer of hope for the future."

In my efforts to reduce the explanation of Chronic Fatigue Syndrome I may have deleted some information that could have been more descriptive but you can see how hard it is to explain the symptoms. Also how different countries vary in their descriptions.

Chapter 2

AUTHOR'S THEORY

Everyone forms an opinion according to observations, research, experience, feelings, etc., so it stands to reason that I would have formed my own opinion, after the extensive research I have undertaken. It may seem controversial to some and thought-provoking to others.

I believe chronic fatigue syndrome may be a result of a catalyst reaction to the central nervous system, perhaps also involving the endocrine system and mostly a change to the gastrointestinal system.

Damaged Adrenal Gland

One theory relates to the adrenal gland not working efficiently and in turn affecting the body's ability to detox, which may have an accumulative effect. This toxic buildup has an effect on liver function, gall bladder, kidneys, hypothalamus, thymus, and the amygdala. I see the endocrine system as our pump, and in CFS sufferers, it's not working well.

Cause of Adrenal Damage

One theory is epinephrine involvement. Synthesized adrenaline is called epinephrine. I believe a reaction between either the quality of the epinephrine manufactured and used worldwide or the amounts of this particular product that we are consuming. It could also be a reaction between synthesized adrenaline to other chemicals that we intake or are exposed to every day.

Explaining the possible damage to the adrenal gland, I use the example of nerve damage (bruised). It takes a very long time to repair and become functional again, of course depending on the damage. If a muscle becomes atrophied and is not working for, say, six weeks, it takes more than three months for it to build up strength again.

So if the endocrine system (the adrenal gland) or the central nervous system becomes bruised or an allergic reaction causes malfunctions with this system, how long would it take the body to repair it?

The adrenal gland that sits on top of the kidneys has our natural adrenaline stores; when they are fatigued, it affects our body all over.

My theory is that because this supply of natural adrenaline is not working properly, it affects the body's ability to detox properly, and the effects are compounded. This is my own unsubstantiated theory and the conclusions I have drawn from research.

Stress

The body is a very sensitive mechanism, and stress or grief or both have also been associated with chronic fatigue syndrome.

Stress is so subtle that sometimes we do not notice we are affected by it, until the particular stress trigger is removed. Then we may say something like "I feel so much better now that we've moved." Or gotten a new job, changed a certain situation, etc. So many times, it is after the fact or event that we notice how much stress we were under.

If our adrenaline glands are pumping out natural adrenaline on a regular basis to deal with stress (emotional/psychological or even environmental, such as hay fever) or the immune system is fighting an infection or disease, such as Epstein-Barr virus, then we introduce a shot of anesthetic with chemical adrenaline (epinephrine) further taxing our immune system. The body's detoxing functioning organs (like our glandular endocrine system) may get tired or overloaded.

I use the analogy of a computer. When you download too many applications, eventually it crashes or freezes.

So after chronic fatigue syndrome develops, we became supersensitive and totally malfunction. I don't have to list the amount of systems like endocrine, digestive, and cognitive that CFS affects.

Anesthetics

Since 1904 when adrenaline was first synthesized, called epinephrine, the medical world has thought it was a good idea to include it in most anesthesia. It seems it made the anesthesia work better and faster. *Faster* is the operative word here.

We also now use adrenaline to treat anaphylactic shock and allergic reactions. The epi pen is the adrenaline pen. This chemical is widely referred to as "adrenaline" outside the United States; however, its United States adopted name and international nonproprietary name is epinephrine. Epinephrine was chosen as the generic name in the United States because John Abel, who prepared extracts from the adrenal glands in 1897, used that name for his extracts.

What do we know about adrenaline?

Long term, what effects does synthesized adrenaline have in the lifetime of a human? Have studies been done on animals as well as humans to determine this? If so, what time span has been monitored? What is a safe quantity and for whom? Is adrenaline safe for everyone? What reactions have people had to this synthesized product? How vigilant have the medical authorities been with accumulating data regarding reactions?

The other big questions are these: Has adrenaline itself changed in the last twenty to forty years? Has there been a better and much-improved adrenaline on the market? Maybe also some cheaper alternatives, compared to the original synthesized adrenaline developed in 1904? It is likely the original composition has changed over the last 110 years. Has the medical market been flooded with cheap substitutes or even added fillers? That may be causing some major allergic reactions or even damage to the adrenal cortex in some people.

Are adrenaline and the hypothalamus inflammation (or overreaction) linked?

Do adrenaline and the immune system have any connections?

The following information is expanding on my theory that anesthetics may be in some way involved in chronic fatigue syndrome.

I feel that anesthetics, in addition to alleviating or blocking out pain, reduce natural adrenaline, a natural product of the adrenal glands that is generally released in association with high stress. Note that adrenaline is also referred to as epinephrine.

So if the slowing release of epinephrine affects and slows the release of oxytocin, which reduces the adrenaline release by adrenal glands, could a reaction (maybe an allergic reaction or intolerance) cause this cycle to get stuck and malfunction, draining the adrenal glands and interfering with the production of natural adrenaline or simply interfering with the natural systemic process?

When did you get chronic fatigue syndrome? After an operation, root-canal therapy, or dental work plus stress caused by any other following?

- grief (death, separation, divorce, or moving house/job/country)
- illness (Epstein-Barr, glandular fever, or any other)
- environmental stress (maybe an allergic reaction)
- emotional stress (too many options to list)
- chemical stress (using a lot of toxic chemicals at a time)

- anything else that lowers the immune system
- food poisoning
- drug, alcohol, or medication

Antihistamines

To clarify my view on antihistamines, I think it's interesting noting the side effects of antihistamine medication—drowsiness, slow reaction time, and difficulty concentrating—that are also some of the chronic fatigue syndrome symptoms.

These symptoms also appear in a person with chronic fatigue syndrome after being exposed to an allergen like paint, after doing too much, or after a stress response.

If the antihistamine's action is to make the body pump through natural adrenaline to get rid of the offending allergen, it could be argued that in chronic fatigue syndrome sufferers, the adrenal gland may be depleted or damaged. The natural adrenaline is disrupted or the pathways are disrupted; therefore, the body does not act normal. It behaves randomly and not at all as we know or are accustomed to seeing body systems act. Therefore, the body is ineffective in detoxing the offending allergen and it stays in high alert, depleting the body of energy.

It's as if the body is having an allergic reaction to its own immune system or an allergen that we have not yet identified.

So Is Poison a Valid Theory?

How does poison affect the body? What are the symptoms? What poisons are possibly consumed? What do we refer to as poison?

Certain substances could be considered poison or foreign to the body. For example, some substances introduced into my body via intravenous administration (preventing my body's natural immune reaction to reject or allow foreign matter). This might include the anesthetics used during caesareans and dental work. They are not used as poison but are foreign to the body. Oral Rohypnol (Flunitrazepam), which is a powerful sedative that depresses the central nervous system, may have been ingested as well.

Symptoms of chemical poisoning for example in respiratory, especially if inhaled, can be stomach cramps, vomiting, and/or diarrhea if the poison was consumed orally and digested into the stomach. Headaches and/or blurry vision you would see from inhaled or accidentally consumed generally these are signs of serious toxicity.

Large amounts of toxic substances in the bloodstream may cause people to show unusual or out-of-character behavior. They may seem listless, confused, or intoxicated. Their movements may also be clumsy or uncoordinated, and the person may complain of dizziness. Chemical poisoning that causes these symptoms should be considered life threatening.

The question I make is this: did my body consider certain substances as poison?

Poison is referred to as a substance that, when introduced into or absorbed by a living organism, causes death or injury, especially one that kills by rapid action, even in a small quantity.

Poison in chemistry is referred to a substance that reduces the activity of a catalyst, in Physics it is referred to as an additive or impurity in a nuclear reactor that slows a reaction by absorbing neutrons.

Under the explanation of poison in chemistry, "a substance that reduces the activity of a catalyst," could there be a link between poison and the body's malfunction? Is poison a plausible reason for the mitochondria malfunction?

Could it be that my mitochondria may not be producing the energy it needs to function in a normal way, causing the body to have a multitude of symptoms as in mitochondria malfunction? Mitochondria function is much better explained by Dr. S. Myhill in the United Kingdom.

Conclusion

There is not one single theory. The glands could be damaged or not acting properly, whether it's the amygdala, adrenal glands, hypothalamus, or the endocrine system as a whole. This could be setting off a whole list of actions and reactions. Was it a poison?

Was it an accumulation of environmental products, plus stress, plus a virus, plus some other weakness? May be or are we having an allergic reaction or an intolerance to the accumulation of anesthetics or the adrenaline in the anesthetics, hard to say.

I do however invite anyone to investigate these theories.

THEORIES BY OTHERS PLUS TREATMENT THEORIES AND IDEAS

Here you will find a few theories that are available today, they make interesting reading and may give you a broader look at Chronic Fatigue Syndrome and Fibromyalgia.

Theory by: Dr Rita Louise, Ph.D.

Chronic Fatigue Syndrome

From Dr. Rita Louise, Ph.D.,

Some health experts believe Chronic Fatigue Syndrome is caused by the Epstein-Barr virus, bronchitis, mononucleosis or hepatitis that goes "underground" and zaps the body of all its resources. Others say that it starts after a period of intense stress, while others believe chronic fatigue is a disease of lifestyle – where we have mismanaged our personal energy resources. And while there are a number of theories as to the origin of this disorder, to date, there is no clear cut definitive cause.

Theory by: Theresa Kelly

The source of this information. Copyright Dewarlorx.com 2007 - Author Theresa Kelly BY Central Sensitivity Syndrome (CSS): Syndrome de Sensibilité Central.

"CSS is a compilation syndrome in which holds overlapping features that can cause significant disability. Such over lapping conditions are Fibromyalgia, myofascial pain, and chronic fatigue syndrome. The biophysiologic mechanisms of these conditions are multifactorial; neuroendocrine abnormalities with central sensitization, however, seem most important. Though psychological distress is present in these patients, keep in mind this is not a psychiatric illness. Management is mostly supportive and includes patient education, psychological support, behavioural modification, physical exercise, and various serotonergic and noradrenergic medications. Like CFS and FMS there is a higher preponderance of females with this condition than men. Accumulated recent data support the hypothesis that all these disorders share a common biophysiologic mechanism of neurohormonal dysregulation caused by perhaps neuroendocrine or adrenaline. It seems the most important neurologic aberrations comprise central sensitization, which involve molecular, chemical, and functional changes in the central nervous system, resulting in an amplification and spread of pain, and intensification of other sensations.

This could be cause by nerve damage, subluxations or inflammation in the central nervous system. One theory in which I have is that damage to the central nervous system causes irritations and inflammation to the blood-brain-barrier and changes its vessel diameter. This change allows chemicals, ions and hormones from the body to enter the brain. These particles are foreign to the brain and thus cause more inflammation and irritation to the rear of the brain such as the medulla oblongata. The medulla is the crossroads for seven major cranial nerves. As these nerves pass through this region of the brain the nerves are excited. Neurotransmitters send the irritative information back down through the central nervous system into the rest of the body. Central sensitization is best described as an amplification and spread of pain due to central nervous system mechanism." www.dewarlorx.com

Theory by: Rolf Gordon.

Geographical stress, this is not a cause but an aggravation. Even though it is explained that if you live long enough over these stress lines or geopathic ley lines you may be susceptible to develop CFS, cancer and other illnesses. www.rolfgordon.co.uk.

Personally I have taken this information and checked my sleeping area, by two different dowsers and Feng Shui experts who came to the same conclusion. My bed was placed over two crossing ley lines, so I moved bedrooms. I have had a recovery of strength and symptoms after this.

Theory by: Dr Paul Cheney

The frequent tachycardias seen with ME/CFS patients have been shown by Dr. Paul Cheney to be a compensatory mechanism that serves to increase cardiac output in the presence of low stroke volume due to diastolic dysfunction in the heart. Orthostatic problems may also be related to diastolic dysfunction as recently shown by Dr. Paul Cheney www.cfids-cab.org.

Theory by: Ian Solley

Ian Solley believes that CFS is related to amalgams. I tend to agree in the sense that amalgams are giving the extra sensitive person (CFS sufferer) a reaction.

I also believe that there are many other forms of reactivity's for CFS sufferers, like underlying infections, allergies and constant exposure, sources of constant stress, whether emotional or physical or chemical, the inability to detox properly giving more symptoms etc as per my theory, under the authors theory section. view his website this cure works.

Theory by: Dr Ashok Gupta

In some information of studies in 2011 showed the hypothesis that the symptoms of ME/CFS/Fibro may be caused by autonomic dysfunction originating in the brain. This is based on comprehensive brain scans of many patients, and is very exciting news and how XMRV retrovirus findings may fit with the amygdala hyperarousal model for ME/CFS.

Recently scientists from the Whittemore Peterson Institute (WPI) led by Dr Mikovits, claim to have discovered a retroviral link to ME/CFS (1). This pioneering research has identified a retrovirus called XMRV, shown to be active in two-thirds of patients (published), and antibodies for the virus were present in 95% of patient (unpublished research).

Mikovits' team said further research must now determine whether XMRV directly causes CFS, is just a passenger virus in the suppressed immune systems of sufferers, or a pathogen that acts in concert with other viruses that have been implicated in the disorder by previous research.

You can read up on more information from Dr Ashok Gupta on www.guptaprogramme.com.

And further, a recent study carried out by Imperial College London attempted to mimic the results of the WPI study (2). They found no evidence of XMRV infection in the blood samples of 186 patients fitting the CDC criteria. They conclude that "Although we found no evidence that XMRV is associated with CFS in the UK, this may be a result of population differences between North America and Europe regarding the general prevalence of XMRV infection, and might also explain the fact that two US groups found XMRV in prostate cancer tissue, while two European studies did not."

The purpose of this paper is to hypothesize how these findings may fit with the Amygdala Hyperarousal Model for ME/CFS (3).

Three Potential Hypotheses

Overall there are three broad hypotheses that we can infer from the findings so far, as per Mikovits' statement:

The XMRV virus directly causes the symptoms of ME/CFS

The XMRV virus indirectly causes ME/CFS by suppressing the immune system in concert with other pathogens, allowing opportunistic viral and bacterial infections to flourish causing the symptoms of ME/CFS

The XMRV virus is simply a passive opportunistic infection which establishes itself due to general suppression and dysfunction of the immune system from another source. (This general immune dysfunction may be caused by autonomic dysfunction as a result of amygdala hyperarousal).

The Amygdala Hyperarousal model states that ME/CFS and Fibromyalgia may be caused by a conditioned trauma in the amygdala following an acute viral, bacterial or physical insult, combined with psycho-social distress. Once the classical and operant conditioning has occurred, the amygdala in association with the insula, become hyper-sensitive to signals from both the body and external stimuli, and magnify both the extent and frequency of the incoming stimuli in the sensory thalamus and cortex. This then produces the ME/CFS vicious circle, where an unconscious sensitivity reaction to symptoms causes chronic stimulation of the HPA axis, immune reactivation/ dysfunction, chronic sympathetic stimulation leading to autonomic dysfunction, mental and physical exhaustion, allergies, compromised detoxification, mitochondria dysfunction, oxidative stress and a host of other distressing symptoms and secondary complications. And these are exactly the symptoms that the amygdala, the insula, and associated limbic structures are trained to monitor and respond to, perpetuating a vicious circle.

(FOR THE FULL ARTICLE PLEASE VIEW www.cfsrecovery.com)

TREATMENT THEORIES AND RECOVERY TOOLS

As you can see there are some theories that are circulating today, my preferred pass time is to concentrate on healing and finding things that work, so I am also including treatment theories.

Harley Johnstone and Dan McDonald (Who can be found on YouTube)

Harley Johnstone explains he experienced healing by A Raw diet (he said he had Crohns Disease and CFS) and Dan McDonald talks about raw food for general strength and wellness and certainly for healing, he talks about the fact that you can heal yourself from many debilitating symptoms. Dan McDonald was my inspiration for going raw. He has a huge amount of material free on YouTube. He also explains that healing and loving yourself come hand in hand, which I tend to agree. This guy is amazing.

TREATMENT IDEAS

Natural Treatments for Epstein-Barr:
www.chronicsorethroat.wordpress.com

An alkalizing diet (or raw food diet) can be effective against Chronic EBV, and for CFS in general. Search for more info on alkalizing/raw food diets. This website explains that alkalizing works because EBV requires acidic tissue conditions to infect certain cells, and therefore alkalizing may go a long way to halting EBV infection. Alkalizing diets also have an anti-inflammatory action, which may also contribute to their healing efficiency.

The following supplements have a useful anti-EBV effect: turmeric, passionflower and sesame seed oil – these inhibit the Epstein-Barr virus. Other anti-EBV supplements include: lysine, ginger, licorice, curcumin, EGCG (from green tea), red marine algae, cayaponia tayuya root, pau d'arco herb, beetroot extract (Beta), olive leaf extract, lemon balm (Melissa officionalis), citrus flavonoids, andrographis paniculata.

MORE TREATMENT THEORIES

Geopathic ley lines and illness is a highly important area that you may like to look into. Research has shown that moving your bed or your bedroom or moving house has had an affect on healing from major illnesses such as cancer and others. If you would like more information check out David Wilcock on GaiamTV, where he has produced several short video presentations on the subject. Also check Kathy Bohler regarding Earth radiation. Search geopathic zones and illnesses.

There is important information, but, judging for yourself is necessary, on Electromagnetic Field(EMF's) and their effect on a sensitive body, like those affected by Chronic Fatigue Syndrome.

EMF exposure may interfere with the body, from detoxing substances like mercury.

EMF exposure may interrupt DNA so it may stop the body from growing and repairing properly.

EMF exposure may interrupt the uptake of melatonin.

You may like to look at earthing your body as a means to personally discharge excessive negative ions and look at your environment and check high readings of EMF's. www.earthingoz.com.au

Finding ways to open your mind and expand your knowledge regarding treatment and theories can be interesting but frustrating as a quick fix pill is not to be found.

Chapter 3

THE GUT

In this section I will be discussing several issues:

Gut bacteria, gut environment, parasites, products and herbs to balance the gut area. The Raw Food Diet is also a very important aspect in the health of the gut.

It is very unusual to find a CFS sufferer without gastrointestinal issues. Whether its constipation, diarrhoea or both, bloating, stomach pain, inflammation, acid build up, heartburn, nausea and others.

Dr Joseph Mercola explains that the gut is where 80% of your immune system is. It has also been referred to as the second brain. That's why when your gut is not functioning well it has an effect on your brain function, psyche and behaviour.

The information on parasites is not new but so very often overlooked. One of the key points with parasites is that their environment needs to be right for them. So if you have an acidic, candida saturated gut they will feel quite at home and love to proliferate in such a comfy setting. It is also common for CFS sufferers to have candida. This comes with sugar cravings, hormonal imbalances, sleep disturbances, brain fog, which I feel can be released with improvement of the gut function.

My first suggestion is to take a gut function test. I was lucky to have met Dr Ian Rafter, Macquarie Street Sydney who tested me to see how my gut was functioning. Based on the results, I was given the special detox diet. As mentioned in the Detox Chapter, it took me about 3 months to master the required 6 weeks nonstop diet requirement. However, once I achieved it, I experienced monumental results.

For the first time my brain fog lifted, and I could read a book again. My memory and my cognitive abilities both improved and I started feeling so much better.

<u>The diet is simple. No wheat, no dairy, and no sugar for six weeks straight, if you break the diet you need to start again.</u>

The reasoning with this is simple - to break the cycle of candida you need to starve the bacteria and parasites by deleting sugar, which is what they feed on.

Wheat turns into sugar, so do carbohydrates, so that's why both need to be kept to a minimum. Wheat also inflames the gut, and dairy produces mucus which candida loves. This environment is perfect for bacteria and parasites. They love this acidic mucusy candida environment, so if you change this environment you will also get rid of the parasites.

There are many other things you can do to assist the expulsion of parasites.

COLONICS

Having colonics on a regular basis is strongly recommended.

There are two different types of colon hydrotherapy available, the close system and the open system. I preferred the open system because it was more like a lounge toilet. I read a book and the practitioner gave me a warm wheat pack for my stomach during the session. The benefits outweigh the stigma of using colonic irrigation.

The closed system is similar but you are on a bed and the practitioner is more involved.

There are bowel cleaning products available such as Dr Hulda Clark's recipes and zapper machine, which I have not tried personally but have heard great reviews for them. I have however used many other types of bowel cleansing products, and there are a few on the market to choose from. I use regularly herbal mixes for parasite control like "Cleanse U" herbal tonic mix. More on detoxes following.

TIPS TO HELP YOU KEEP THE GOOD BACTERIA IN YOUR GUT AREA

Eat fermented foods e.g. Sauerkraut.Keifer

Pickled fermented foods like cabbage, turnips, eggplant, onions, and carrots.

Taking probiotics, and there are a few on the market to choose from.

Regarding Helicobacter pylori problems in the gut an interesting advice from Dr Michael T Murray was to drink cabbage juice for 10 days look up Dr Mercola's website www.mercola.com.

With other digestive problems e.g. irritable bowel syndrome, ulcerative colitis, celiac disease, diarrhoea and constipation, improvement from these diseases lies in: the understanding of enzymes and probiotics.

Improving your digestive health naturally with an anti-inflammatory diet raw food, and lifestyle.

An interesting point, the gut has ten times more microbial species than the overall amount of cells in the entire body. These microbial bacterial, (often called good bacteria) break down food into small nutrients that are absorbed in the gut into the bloodstream. They also help to detoxify the body and help in the immunity functions, like in the case of food poisoning. If the ratio of these bacteria is too low it causes chronic inflammation therefore leading to digestive problems.

Clean water is essential for good health. Most people drink water containing chlorine a disinfectant by-product and other environmental toxins. As you drink chlorinated water it will also sterilize the body by destroying progenic cultures. The body is susceptible to opportunistic pathogenic species such as candida.

The ultimate water to drink would be from a natural spring; it is the most bio energetically alive water and often contains healthy bacteria and is also generally alkaline.

Reverse osmosis filtration works well and there are a number of systems on the market. One that I have tested personally is the Genzon water system which was inspired by Dr Emoto's work. I have tested the water and it has a good PH balance. Also note adding freshly squeezed lemon or apple cider vinegar to your water is another idea to add anti-oxidant properties to it and help with alkalinity in the body, a very important aspect of the gut function and its connection to leaky gut syndrome.

Following is some advice from: www.crohns.net.

Leaky Gut Syndrome is not a disease but an intestinal dysfunction that can underlie many different illnesses and symptoms. It can be caused by poor food choices, insufficient pancreatic digestive enzymes, chronic stress, environmental contaminants, gastrointestinal disease, immune overload, too much alcohol, dysbiosis, and longtime use of NSAIDs (non-steroidal, anti-inflammatory drugs). NSAID's, steroids, antacids, and antibiotics are probably the greatest contributors to leaky gut syndrome. Birth Control pills and steroid drugs exacerbate the situation. Chemo-drugs and radiation therapy can also disrupt GI tract balance significantly.

I found the release of the "brain fog" symptom was so significant with my own experience as well as other symptoms of CFS such as the bloated stomach and the nausea that even though the body pain and the heavy feeling in the body persisted, having a significant change in these symptoms gave me the strength to contemplate seriously that CFS may one day be taking a back seat in my health. I researched and held tightly the belief that improving gut function and leaky gut syndrome would produce great results for CFS symptoms.

Views on Leaky Gut Syndrome:

Inflamed gastro intestinal tract is associated with leaky gut syndrome.

The gut does not absorb nutrients and foods properly so it may result in fatigue and bloating.

When the detoxification pathways that line the gut are compromised, chemical sensitivities may occur. (This is why I believe that Colonics is so important)

The leaking of toxins also burdens the liver so that the body is less able to handle everyday chemicals.

Carrier proteins may also be damaged so nutrient deficiencies occur which may cause a variety of symptoms, like magnesium deficiency (connected to muscle spasms and fibromyalgia) copper deficiency leads to high cholesterol and osteoarthritis, zinc deficiency leads to malabsorption which causes hair loss and some eye disorders, and may also be related to depression.

When the gut lining is inflamed it is believed that the body is unable to ward off bacteria, viruses and parasites as well as fungus and yeast like candida. These pathogens then pass from the gut cavity to the bloodstream and set up infection anywhere else in the body.

(This could be an important theory, regarding loss of energy for the CFS sufferer; because the body is constantly having to deal with underlying infections in the body it takes up a lot of energy to fight infections)

The formation of antibodies may occur as they leak across and could possibly look similar to antigens on our own tissue. So they could be attacked by the body thinking it is foreign material. They believe this could be a possibility on how Crohns disease, Lupus, rheumatoid arthritis and multiple sclerosis start.

So the combination of these actions encourage the formation of toxins, the toxins can also leak into the system, so when food particles escape through then it could leak into the blood stream, the immune system senses that they are a threat (body produces antigens to combat this) and it results in food sensitivities.

Some of the noted symptoms of Leaky gut are confusion, memory loss and brain fog, as well as food allergies and sensitivities.

Usually the bacteria fungi and parasites would not be able to go through the barrier of the gut.

These lovely creatures and their toxins are usually present in large amounts and can overwhelm the liver's ability to detoxify. Important point here, this is why I feel it is very important to do a liver detox.

Other products and foods that can have a negative effect on this already bad situation are taking antibiotics, drinking alcohol and coffee (they greatly irritate the gut).

Foods that have bacteria or parasites like giardia lamblia, crystopsporidium, blastocystis hominis, also helicobacter pylori, klebsiella, citrobacter, pseudomonas and others.

Chemicals in processed foods, dyes, preservatives, peroxidised fats (using the same oil over and over).

My Note: (Oxidised rancid oil combined with a couple of vodkas had sent me to hospital with a gall bladder attack. The liver will not love you for it. Like in my case. Interesting also to note here is that I was emotionally upset at a situation at the time. I believe anger, sadness, grief could be triggers for a gallbladder upset.

Having an enzyme deficiency, similar in people with celiac disease, lactose deficiency for those with lactose intolerance.

NSAIDS (non-steroidal anti-inflammatory drugs) like neurophen, ibuprofen, indomethacin, Mobic, Celebrex, Brufen, Naprosyn, Orudis and Voltaren.

Corticosteroids like Prednisone, Hydrocortisone, Depomedrol.

Refined carbohydrate diet like cakes, cookies, white bread, soft drinks, chocolate bars, etc.

Prescription hormones like the contraception pill.

Mould and fungal mycotoxins in stored grain, fruit and refined carbohydrates.

Chemo-therapy and radiation therapy causing immune overload.

Symptoms of inflammation of the gastro intestinal tract, associated with leaky gut syndrome view Dr Liz Lipski www.lizlipski.com.

HERBS

The herbal composition that can assist with a leaky gut state, of the gastro intestinal tract area I found useful was "CleanseU," this tonic mix was developed by Eli Shammon in Parramatta, NSW, Australia. It has the following actions: liver cleanse, intestinal cleanse, fluid retention, constipation, intestinal worms, parasites, digestive disorders, bowel health, weight management and flatulence.

CleanseU contains the following herbal ingredients: Cloves relieves worms, viruses, candida, and various bacterial and protozoan infestations Wormwood expels intestinal worms, relieves digestive disorders Black Walnut expels intestinal worms; antimicrobial and anti-fungal effects Alfalfa aids digestion and nutrient assimilation Cayenne aids digestion; this tonic has many more herbs and the combination is what I believe has an amazing healing effect specific for people with Chronic Fatigue Syndrome.

A very important message for gut function is to attend to parasites, intestinal parasites, says Barbara Bryant, which can thrive in your body regardless of your living conditions or location. They can cause illnesses ranging from chronic fatigue syndrome to cancer. Cloves kill parasitic eggs and when used in conjunction with black walnut tincture and wormwood, the combination can rid the body of at least 100 varieties of parasites.

A Naturopath will be able to recommend herbal tonics for gut function support. The Australian association is the Australian Traditional Medicine Society in Sydney where you can find a registered practitioner.

EXERCISE: CONSCIOUS EATING

Aim to eat like the monks.

If you are eating fast. Stop.

Breathe in for the count of 2 – hold 1 and exhale 2.

Hold for the count of 2 – 1 and 2

Breathe out for the count of 2 – 1 and 2 repeat this until you feel your body relax and your mind slows down.

Make sure your body is centered.

Spend a minute or two centering yourself.

The gut is sensitive to stimuli and the central nervous system therefore you have a better chance at digestion when you are calm.

EXERCISE: CENTERING

How to centre yourself, your energy, your body.

Step one: Stop breathing for a few seconds. Hold your breath and release. You can do this several times to find your balance.

Step two: Tune into your body. Notice how your body is vibrating. Notice if any part of the body is vibrating differently, e.g. your head might be thumping and your finger tips numb.

Step three: Do the breathing exercise

Breathe in for the count of 2 – 1 and 2

Hold for the count of 2 – 1 and 2

Breathe out for the count of 2 – 1 and 2 repeat this until your feel your body relax and your mind slow down.

Option 1: Sometimes we have too much built up energy or nervous energy and we need to clear it out so we can balance the breath and the nervous system with the following:

Step: Breath in 1,2, then hold 1,2, then breath out forcefully, repeat 2 or 3 times or as necessary.

Option 2: There are times when you feel sluggish and sedated, you don't feel like moving much or your body may have been in the same position for too long. In this case try the following:

Step: Breathe in deeply then breathe out. Next take a bigger breath, then breathe out. Next take a deep breath and hold then breath in again to put more air in the lungs then out and continue to breath normal. So as to extend the lungs just that little extra.

EXERCISE: STOMACH AND CORE

Many times when a muscle has been overused, cramped or in spasm for long periods of time it becomes fatigued and "turned off." To activate this muscle again you need to release it. Following are a few ways of re-activating the muscle or releasing and relaxing the muscles.

Do the Cat and Dog stretch, taught by Yoga teachers. Take a yoga class to get this stretch correctly. If you cannot attend a class view the instructions on YouTube. How to Do a yoga cat cow pose for energy.

Do a positional release or a (PNF)proprioceptive neuromuscular facilitation or (met) muscle energy technique release, if you could attend a registered remedial massage therapist treatment ask if they do these releases when you go for a massage.(ATMS is the association in Australia) A brief description of this treatment as follows: the practitioner will place their hand on the belly of the muscle, the abs (abdominus) for example where the muscle is most weak and then ask you to breath in as you breath out you push your stomach out on to the hand of the practitioner and release the breath, this technique is done not more than 3 times on one particular area, as it can be painful, during or the next day. Allow time for recovery I prefer 2 weeks, then have another treatment with the remedial massage practitioner until you feel that the muscles of your stomach are turning on and off correctly.

You can also get a Kinesiologist to test what muscles need more attention. For example abdominus erectus or obliques or transverse.

Visit a Pilates trainer and preferably attend a one on one session with the objective to learn breathing exercises and core strength work, to activate this area from the inside. This will help to stimulate the under-active interior muscles and body structures such as ligaments and tendons and release the tight areas and bring balance to the gut area.

There is an important need to balance. So attend to the upper back between the shoulder blades, these muscles are called the rhomboids.

This exercise is done by yourselves and sitting in a straight up right position then placing your thoughts in the middle of your upper back squeeze together the shoulder blades tightly for a count of 10 then release. 3 times for 3 days. Keeping shoulders neck and arms relaxed. Do this for the first week, then again the next week for 3 weeks. Monitor how you are feeling. Then as necessary, my recommendation is once per week for 6 months and depending how weak the muscles are, is how much stomach work you are doing. Always balance this exercise with the stomach muscles exercises.

Note: these kinesiology techniques and massage techniques will be taught on the workshops and training on my website. www.chronicfatigueshop.com.au.

Another exercise for the stomach area is to stimulate it by tapping. Hold your breath and hold the muscles of your stomach hard for a few minutes and tap the abdominal muscles with your fingertips.

Chakra healing of the solar plexus, with a practitioner or a Reiki master you will balance the energy in the solar plexus. Read more detail on this centre under the Healing chapter.

Wear clothes with the colour orange, and visualize the colour orange on your stomach area as you hold the thought of "already healed."

Affirmation to use with and during all of these exercises. Thank you for my healing, I feel strong, powerful and centered now. I am sorry please forgive me for ignoring. I love you (insert your name). You will find clarification on these exercises in the workshops and training available on www.chronicfatigueshop.com.au

Below are some other suggestions that may help to activate a weak abdominal area.

Tapping on the stomach area minimum of 50 taps, a gentle technique using rhythm with the tips of your fingers gently tap onto the abdominal muscles for a count of 50 taps.

Using a Tens machine and attach the pads to the abdominal area. A physiotherapist clinic usually has these machines for sale, the cost in Australia is usually around $150, and you can also find them online and on eBay. I have now tried this personally and can see how this can tighten and activate weak stomach muscles as well as pump out possible toxins through the lymph system and nodes of the abdominal muscles.

I recommend reading Leaky Gut syndrome by Dr Liz Lipski (www.innovativehealing.com) it is a small book costing $3.95. LEAKY GUT BOOK BY DR LIZ LIPSKY: This mechanism comes into play in Chronic Fatigue Syndrome. The cells are screaming for nutrients, the immune system is on overdrive, and the digestive system is not working adequately. When digestive mechanisms come back into balance, the body's innate healing capacity is enhanced. Dysbiosis is a term that identifies an imbalance in the 300-400 normal types of bacteria normally found in our intestinal tracts. New research indicates that some auto-immune diseases, like lupus disease, rheumatoid arthritis, and ankylosing spondilitis, have both bacterial and genetic components. When a person with a specific genetic make-up meets the wrong bacteria, conditions are ideal for auto-immune disarray.

Using fermented foods to improve gut function, during the fermentation the plant ingredients being fermented by the beneficial microorganisms are broken down or pre-digested. This makes the nutrients in these plants more easily digested and absorbed by your body and daily consumption of the fermented foods also improves the balance of your intestinal flora. Fermented foods are naturally rich in enzymes which further support your digestive system.

You can buy digestive enzymes at the health food store and some pharmacies. As well as probiotics. Read Dr Mercolas website and his recommendations on "tips for optimizing gut bacteria."

RAW FOODS

My personal success with eating raw foods.

Raw foods have all the natural enzymes to naturally break down food making digestion easy and nutrients absorption in its ultimate state or facilitation. If the gastro intestinal tract is inflamed as it usually is with chronic fatigue sufferers and allergies or abundant intolerances, eating raw foods will help to clear out and sooth inflammation and rid you of built up glue like sediment from the gastro intestinal area. It is best to achieve 90% to 98% raw consumption for the length of time that you desire.

The alkaline diet is also best for gut function. Alkaline forming foods are safe foods to eat. Rest and sleep are alkaline builders. Stress is acid forming. Exercise is alkaline forming, breathing fresh air, pleasure, laughter, enjoyment and love are alkaline forming. Acid forming are worry, fear, anger, gossip, hatred, envy, selfishness, and even silence. We are what we eat, mentally we are what we think and spiritually we are what we believe. Visit www.jbsoulscan.com/content/acid-alkaline-diet-food-chart.

My suggestion is to look up and study carefully what the alkaline diet is about, and study the chart. Please note that there are foods that are acidic but turn alkaline when they are consumed.

Coconut water and coconut milk, raw coconuts. The water from coconuts is antibacterial and antiviral it is a very wholesome food as well as a healing food. There is much information on the benefits of coconuts available online and I highly recommend you research this area.

Dr Hulda Clark, and the Zapper machine for parasite and bacterial control. This is an amazing lady who has dedicated herself to detoxing, she has a lifetime dedication worth of material to help people heal from parasites and bacteria, she has developed many different types of cleanses. Visit huldaclarkzappers website.

Honey: Raw honey, I use regularly as an antibacterial for flu viruses in particular and can be used not only internally but also externally, any fungus or for bugs on the skin, I like Manuka honey from New Zealand.

Zeolite powder: a mud like substance is very helpful for bacteria and viruses, I like using this by sprinkling some in a glass of water and gargling for sore throats, mouth ulcers, bad breath, white coated tongue to name a few. This clay is known for absorbing chemicals but it works well in neutralizing odours and some studies suggest benefits with bacteria and viruses. I use this every day, one of my favourites.

Chapter 4

DETOX

I view detoxing as a priority for a chronic fatigue syndrome sufferer, as the central nervous system and the lymphatic system may not be working well. The detoxing organs may also not be functioning well: the liver, gallbladder, kidneys, thymus, thyroid, lymphatic nodules and the spleen. The endocrine system is so affected, it's overwhelmed.

One of the viruses that can affect the spleen for example is Epstein Barr Virus and other infectious mononucleosis. These have being shown to have an association with people suffering chronic fatigue syndrome. It's not known whether one of these viruses are present before or after, the symptoms of chronic fatigue syndrome present, or whether there is a direct link between viruses and this illness.

I have found that the central nervous system is so overactive that it may affect the endocrine system, the hormones, the sleeping patterns, the brain, the muscles and the heart in a way that is disruptive.

Calming the central nervous system is the KEY.

This can be achieved using, will power, meditation, detoxing, breathing techniques and of course I found the Amygdala Retraining

Program invaluable. This system developed by Ashok Gupta in the UK helps to retrain your reactions and therefore has a direct effect on the central nervous system. As a Kinesiologist I connected and understood this technique and I have taken the technique on board wholeheartedly.

The immune system generally is strongest when we have removed the accumulation of toxins, yeast, bacteria, drugs and other irritating substances from our body. Restoring vitamins and minerals by eating nutrient dense whole foods, real foods, makes sense to me, so, ultimately, raw food.

The function of the immune system is to protect the body and maintain a good barrier against infections, bacteria, viruses, yeast, toxins and other self-damaging cells like cancer cells so detoxing is a good way of increasing energy and strength.

The immune system is made up of our bone marrow, the thymus gland, the lymph nodes, the spleen, tonsils, adenoids and the appendix. These glands and organs develop lymphocytes, which are the white cells, the worker cells of the immune system. The primary lymphocytes are B-cells, T-cells, natural killer cells, macrophages and dendritic cells.

So one of the keys to keeping the immune system strong is to detox and cleanse our body. I like using raw fruit and vegetables for this purpose, so plenty of juices, salads and smoothies.

Detoxing means a 90% to 98% raw diet, maintenance is anything below that.

Zeolite powder, as a chemical detox tool, is fantastic and colonics are also recommended.

Why exactly do we need to detox? Firstly, let's review the everyday pollutants so we can then address and understand the need for detoxing the body.

FOOD POISONING

Food poisoning apparently is very common. For most people it is usually mild, but food poisoning can be severe and even terminal for some individuals.

Cases of food poisoning occur when people eat food or drink water containing bacteria, bacterial toxins (substances produced by bacteria), parasites, or viruses. Food poisoning can also occur when non-infectious poisons (such as poisonous mushrooms) or heavy metals (such as lead or mercury) are ingested or injected into the blood stream.

Check out what medication or vaccines use as preservatives. If you use the flu vaccine ask your naturopath what things you can do prior to taking the flu shot to enhance or protect your immune system beforehand.

It is estimated that about 11 million Canadians experience food poisoning each year, and the Food safety Information Council, Australia, estimates 5 million Australians experience food poisoning each year and approximately 120 people die. (Food standards Australia and New Zealand).

People at greatest risk for food poisoning are seniors, pregnant women, young children and babies, and people with chronic medical conditions (e.g., diabetes, AIDS, liver disease) I feel chronic fatigue syndrome sufferers should also be in this category.

Some Causes of Food Poisoning

Food poisoning occurs when contaminated food or water is ingested. Contamination can occur anywhere along the process of obtaining and eating food. It can happen during the growing, harvesting, processing, storing, or preparation stages. In most cases, bacteria, viruses, or parasites are transferred to food from other sources, making these organisms the most common causes of food poisoning. However, in some less common types of food poisoning, the poison or toxin is naturally part of the food (e.g. poisonous mushrooms or fish). Other less common causes include shellfish and insecticides.

Bacteria and bacterial toxins: Many bacteria can cause food poisoning, either directly or by the toxins they produce. Some of the most common include Salmonella, E. coli, Shigella, Staphylococcus, and Clostridium perfringens. Many bacterial causes of food poisoning are due to undercooked meats, poultry, eggs, dairy, processed meats, fish, custards, cream pies, and contaminated water.

Viruses: Norovirus and other viruses can cause food poisoning. Most commonly through contaminated, raw or uncooked produce and shellfish from contaminated water.

Parasites: Parasites such a giardia lamblia can also cause food poisoning through contaminated produce and water.

A good friend of mine's youngest child contracted giardia when he was in preschool and her child's eating habits from then on changed. He has only been able to tolerate a small selection of foods since then.

With parasitic poisoning, once you have experienced this, the body develops a memory and the bodies shock response from being so sick takes a long time to repair, giardia, for example.

Mushrooms, fish and shellfish can contain toxic levels of contamination.

Also we need to remember that these fish are susceptible to all the toxins in the oceans and water ways, which are being bombarded with pollution. The pesticides and insecticides that we dump in our water ways or get dragged down with rains and storms. Nuclear disasters, oil spills etc.

Insecticides: There are many types of poisons found in insecticides but the most dangerous types are the organophosphates, which are basically nerve gas for insects.

There are many other causes of food poisoning. These include wild nuts, leaves, flowers and berries, botulism bacteria, cadmium from containers, lead or arsenic from fertilizers, and acids and lead from pottery.

NOTE:
Just to note whenever I come in contact with fertilizers I have a CFS reaction, my body goes weak, I become cranky, headaches, body ache, fogginess, what seems to work for me is taking an anti-histamine and lie down without a pillow under my head for as long as it takes for

my body to stop reacting. I drink plenty of water and do some deep breathing exercises.

Pesticide poisoning:

Too many to list so I chose one: Organophosphate and carbamate insecticides, and below are some of the symptoms:
Signs and symptoms associated with mild exposures to organophosphate and carbamate insecticides include:
Headache, fatigue, dizziness, loss of appetite with nausea, stomach cramps and diarrhoea;
Blurred vision associated with excessive tearing;
Contracted pupils of the eye;
Excessive sweating and salivation;
Slowed heartbeat, often fewer than 50 per minute;
Rippling of surface muscles just under the skin.

These symptoms may be mistaken for those of flu, heat stroke or heat exhaustion, or upset stomach.

Moderately severe organophosphate and carbamate insecticide poisoning cases exhibit all the signs and symptoms found in mild poisonings, but also the person may experience:
Unable to walk;
Often complains of chest discomfort and tightness;
Exhibits marked constriction of the pupils (pinpoint pupils);
Exhibits muscle twitching;
Has involuntary urination and bowel movement.

Cadmium found in pesticides is one of the chemicals with interesting side effects.

For this book, I have chosen Cadmium. After having a hair analysis, this particular chemical was very high in my own body's test readings and geographically where I lived the people associated with having CFS have also come up with Cadmium in their hair analysis. View for more details. Inter Clinical Laboratories Pty Ltd. (hair analysis) Australia www.interclinical.com.au

Some places where we could find this chemical:

Smelting works and refining of metals, batteries, plastic coatings, art paint: oranges, reds and yellows in chalk, and pastels, phosphate in fertilizers.

What is Cadmium?

Cadmium is a by-product of the mining and smelting of lead and zinc. It is used in nickel-cadmium batteries, PVC plastics, and paint pigments. It can be found in soils because insecticides, fungicides, sludge, and commercial fertilizers that use cadmium are used in agriculture.

Cadmium may be found in reservoirs containing shellfish. Cigarettes also contain cadmium.

Lesser-known sources of exposure are dental alloys, electroplating, motor oil, and exhaust. Inhalation accounts for 15-50% of absorption through the respiratory system; 2-7% of ingested cadmium is absorbed in the gastrointestinal system. Target organs are the liver, placenta, kidneys, lungs, brain, and bones.

Due to the bodies sensitivities, there could be many things that affect you now, in which did not affect you before, therefore I would suggest you may like to take this information to your Naturopath for discussion and a possible hair analysis test.View www.lef.org/protocols.

Clinical effects of Cadmium:

"Acute exposure to cadmium fumes may cause flu like symptoms including chills, fever, and muscle ache sometimes referred to as "the cadmium blues."

Symptoms may resolve after a week if there is no respiratory damage. More severe exposures can cause trachea-bronchitis, pneumonitis, and pulmonary edema. Symptoms of inflammation may start hours after the exposure and include cough, dryness and irritation of the nose and throat, headache, dizziness, weakness, fever, chills, and chest pain.

Please research cadmium if you feel it relates to your symptoms.

In my particular case the high cadmium readings within my body is being addressed by my Naturopath with homeopathics and herbal tonic Cleanse U. As well, I take care of my kidneys by drinking clean alkaline water, green tea, raw parsley in my tea as well as Zeolite powder daily.

"The association of symptoms indicative of acute toxicity is not difficult to recognize because the symptoms are usually severe, rapid in onset, and associated with a known exposure or ingestion (Ferner 2001): cramping, nausea, and vomiting; pain; sweating; headaches; difficulty breathing; impaired cognitive, motor, and language skills; mania; and convulsions. The symptoms of toxicity resulting from chronic exposure (impaired cognitive, motor, and language skills;

learning difficulties; nervousness and emotional instability; and insomnia, nausea, lethargy, and feeling ill) are also easily recognized; however, they are much more difficult to associate with their cause. Symptoms of chronic exposure are very similar to symptoms of other health conditions and often develop slowly over months or even years. Sometimes the symptoms of chronic exposure actually abate from time to time, leading the person to postpone seeking treatment, thinking the symptoms are related to something else." view website lef.org/protocols.

Now about those symptoms, they sound way too familiar, could they be described as: brain fog, headaches, sleeping problems, gastrointestinal problems and body pain and lets not forget lethargy and tiredness, I am certainly not implying that Chronic Fatigue Syndrome is cadmium poisoning but I am making a connection with poisoning in general.

A connection I feel worthy of exploring: When the body is under emotional stress, e.g., grieving and a physiological stress of an underlying infection e.g. Epstein Barr, something like going to the dentist (or having an operation) when the body is injected with anesthetic (which contains synthetic adrenaline), or maybe a severe allergic reaction to some product or allergic stimulant, (a combination of these or an accumulation of these), in my opinion could have a connection in disrupting the body, causing a "chronic fatigue syndrome," functioning body.

In my opinion, the CNS, (central nervous system), becomes depleted and unable to function normally. It becomes disorganized, affecting all other systems, endocrine, cardiac, immune, lymphatic.

NOTE: After researching how other people have recovered from chronic fatigue syndrome, it is clear, that detoxifying plays a major part. I not only observed the results from detoxifying combined with a raw food diet, I believe it has healed my gastrointestinal tract and by alkalinizing my blood it has had a huge beneficial effect on my symptoms of CFS.

WHAT YOU CAN DO?

Detoxing your body is one of the best ways to begin the process of taking care of your health. Most people understand the importance of detoxing as our lifestyle has become increasingly more complicated. Following is a basic list for detoxing.

Things to Eliminate:

Polluted water replaced with Filtered Water

Removing chemicals from home

Removing fragrances

Buying safe washing powder

Using chemical free shampoo and conditioners

Make up, using safe mineral make up without nasty chemicals. (Use the lipstick and gold ring test: rub a gold ring on your lipstick mark on the back of your hand and if it turns black it may contain lead or lead traces).

Hand wash or soap: Use Zeolite mineral soap instead or to cancel out the chemicals straight zeolite powder.

Kitchen: remove non-stick frying pans and silicone baking trays and plastics of all kinds.

All chemical cleaning products. Use vinegar, bicarb soda and zeolite powder (great for cleaning metal pots).

At work: e.g. carpenters or upholsterers using very toxic glues could use Zeolite soap, wear a mask do not inhale arsenic dipped timber shavings for example.

At the office: fumes from liquid paper, toner, ink, etc.

Wash all fruit and vegetables with a spoon of apple cider vinegar, preferable buy organic.

Toilet: make sure you move your bowels every day. (Enemas or colonics, change diet, fibre etc.)

Drinking plenty of water everyday not sometimes.

Exercise is a form of detoxing, the lactic acid that forms in the muscles can move through the lymphatic fluid powered by exercise.

Infra-red saunas are another form of detoxing.

Removing herbicides and pesticides and heavy metals from the body. Try Zeolite powder.

Bowel cleansing is very important because we eat plenty of questionable additives, not only chemicals but also parasites. "CleanseU" is a herbal tonic that can help with this.

There are other elimination diets for example, like the anti-candida diet.

Other singular herbs and homeopathic too can be used to eliminate certain toxins.

Bi-carb soda used daily, in things like brushing your teeth, drinking a glass of water with a tea spoon of bi-carb. This helps to change the internal environment where viruses and bacteria live.

Language: Detoxing negative, destructive language from everyday use. The body becomes weak when it is engaged in a large percentage of negative language therefore the opposite can also have a major affect. Positive language is a necessity and is essential for a chronic fatigue syndrome sufferer. (View work on Dr Emoto's research regarding water changes).

THINGS THAT CAN MAKE THE BODY WEAK

Aspartame: this product has other names also, artificial sweetener.

MSG: natural or synthesized or flavour enhancer (chips, packet food, etc)

Yeast overgrowth: Do a test. Delete sugar/bread from your diet. (Note: inflammation in the gut equals inflammation in the brain).

Note: I like my coffee, but I took it out of my diet during my intensive 2 month raw diet cleanse. And now I can have a coffee here and there without too much bother to my energy levels.

Caffeine (burns out the adrenal gland and causes inflammation)

Gluten: is a protein in wheat. Immune system reacts and could become inflamed: There are no symptoms most of the time, unless you have been tested for coeliac.

Dairy: Major protein, if you have a possible leaky gut you can have a reaction to diary. Butter or Ghee is sometimes ok.

Soy: Soy protein and leaky gut symptoms do not mix (soy lethesin may be ok) check out Liz Lipski on www.innovativehealing.com she talks about leaky gut syndrome and has loads of information.

The Lymphatic System: Your bodies personal detox system.

Lymph fluid plus cellular fluids are what makes up a large percentage of body fluid. All nutrients, oxygen, carbon dioxide and other metabolic by-product waste travel from each of our billions of cells, carried by lymph fluid.

Lymph fluid can either be reabsorbed into the blood, or be filtered by one or more lymph nodes before re-entering the bloodstream.

When it's not working efficiently, the lymphatic system reduces the ability for the brain and other organs to do their work. Toxins normally filtered out and destroyed by the lymph system are offloaded onto other organs, like the liver or kidneys, which may overload them in some circumstances.

Similar to what happens in the intestine and colon with poor health and nutritional habits, a stagnant lymph fluid may contain old deposits of dead bacteria, metabolic toxins, and dead cells.

Looking at what things can influence the lymphatic system negatively:

Overworking and taking little time for rest;

An inactive lifestyle, doing very little movement or exercise;

Processed foods and restricted intake of fresh/raw foods;

Chronic depression, negative language/thoughts

Toxic chemical-based pollutants

Energy blocks, attitudes and behaviours. Stiff, blocked thinking, stubborn

Restricting spirituality or concentrating too much on material aspects of life.

When the lymph system becomes blocked or sluggish, a toxic environment may be created which may influence all the cells of the body. A stagnant toxic lymph flow could produce a thickened, dirty lymph, instead of the liquid being more fluid. It may have a degeneration effect of cells and organs. It has been shown that consistent improvement following lymph drainage massage or other lymph clearing processes is experienced.

My lymphatic system changed when I started detoxing and even more when I started eating a raw diet. As a massage therapist I pay a lot of attention to skin and lymphatic flow and I noticed my skin texture improve and became soft, smooth, tighter, especially under my arms, between the creases of the arms and legs, ankles, wrists and most noticeably my neck, which reduced in size (about one and a half inches).

It is very important to note that when a client is experiencing acute symptoms of CFS, like headaches, aching body and muscles and not feeling well, massage for a full hour can have a contra-indicated effect on the symptoms. That is, it is best to have a massage when you are feeling the strongest at the time not the weakest. Because it will push all the toxins around and you will experience an increase in symptoms and then the body has to work hard to detox the excess toxins that have been moved by the massage.

I feel that getting a treatment on your neck for example is enough, then make another appointment to deal with another area of the body and pace your massage treatments.

You may benefit from lymphatic detoxing if you suffer from any of the following;

Back pain
Breast congestion
Chronic bowel problems e.g.. Constipation
Yeast infections
Chronic fatigue syndrome
Fibromyalgia
Skin disorders
Cellulite fat accumulations
Rheumatoid arthritis
Chemical sensitivities
Hormonal and emotional imbalances

Recurrent headaches
Chronic depression
Muscle and tissue tension
Chronic sinusitis, allergies
Gum disease and bad breath
Hearing, balance or sight problems
Re-occurring tonsillitis, colds,
Prostatitis or other glandular problems
Overweight
Lupus
Hemorrhoids
Slow healing burns or cuts.

Detox and Cleansing:

It is important to take responsibility for your own life, which includes health. However, we are all individuals, and we all have to find our own way and what works best for us.

There is a wealth of information on alternative and complementary medicine, including internal cleansing and detoxing. Below are a few cleanses developed by Hulda R. Clark. I highly recommend you read some of her books. Her work is brilliant. I recommend her teas.

I cannot stress enough how important I believe detoxing is for chronic fatigue syndrome, fibromyalgia and chemical sensitivities sufferers.

Following is a list of other cleanses:

Bacteria Cleansing: Eliminating toxic bacteria from the stomach and the gastro intestinal system, infections and food poisoning.

Blood Cleansing: Cleansing the blood can help to lower cholesterol and reduce cardiovascular incidents as well as arterial lesions and vein wall health. Pay attention to liver flushes which can help with blood cleansing.

Candida Cleansing: Controlling the over population of candida albicans. Try to eliminate sugar from your diet for 2 months.

Colon Cleanse: There are colon cleanses done professionally as well as enemas which you can do at home, you can buy an enema kit on line or through some pharmacies.

Heavy Metal Cleanse: Eliminating heavy metals and environmental toxins. There are therapies like Chelation Therapy, Bio-resonance, CH7 homeopathic heavy metal detox, as well as herbal heavy metal detox. Zeolite powder detox for heavy metals, (my favourite).

Kidney Cleanse: Cleaning your filters is vital. The kidneys also sit right under the adrenal glands (supposedly the malfunctioning organ for chronic fatigue sufferers). Don't forget bladder and gallbladder. Using a few leaves of fresh parsley in your water is brilliant for your kidneys.

Liver cleaning: There are some great products out there for liver cleansing, mostly herbal formulas, tablets, powders and tonics.

Parasite Cleansing: Eliminating parasites mostly with a herbal preparation. I use "CleanseU," a herbal tonic in Australia developed by Naturopath Eli Shammon.

I have used CleanseU, which is also called Herbal Detox Tonic, for many years now, and can recommend this product. Eli Shamon has helped many thousands of people in a very ill predicament.

Important: Some other ways of cleansing, especially through the lymphatic system, is exercise, movement, pumping and massaging the body, Saunas and spas.

DETOXING WITH ENEMAS

With enemas you can prevent the accumulation of constipated waste in the lower bowel. Your blood will begin to clean-up right away. When this happens the toxins that are concentrated in your tissues will diffuse back into the blood where they will be eliminated by your liver and kidneys. Your liver and kidneys are no longer overwhelmed by toxins and as long as you control constipation and try to avoid pollution from other sources, your liver and kidneys can do an amazing job.

Many serious diseases may be avoided through this gentle, scientific technique. Enemas are a key factor in the restoration of the body's natural balance and overall health. It can be helpful in any type of ailment, like headache, fever etc. Enemas should be kept to a minimum and used only for short periods. They are not meant to replace a healthy bowel movement and prolonged use will make the colon lazy.

DETOXING WITH COLONICS

Colonics or Colon Hydrotherapy is generally the cleansing of the large intestine with water. Also referred to as bathing as it implies a much nicer and gentler procedure.

This is done by letting approximately 60 liters of water washing the colon during a period of approximately forty-five minutes.

The colon is about 150 cm to 170 cm long. It is important to cleanse all of it. The special equipment used will enable this process. Colonics, unlike enemas, should have no internal pressure and therefore have no discomfort. If you have a lot of gas you can experience slight cramping during the colonics which is usually short lived as the gas leaves the colon. The colon is stimulated by this method.

A colonic removes a lot more than an enema, the process is gentle but very effective.

A view tube is available for observation, usually and all matter is eliminated into the sewage, there are no smells etc. You do nothing but lie back and relax with an open system colonic. The main difference between an open system colonic and a closed system colonic session is that the therapist will be with you from the beginning to end, explaining everything to you and attending to your needs during the session. The therapist will give you a deep belly massage to help eliminate waste from the colon. As the nerves of the colon respond to the soles of your feet your therapist will also manipulate and stimulate the colon reflexes in your feet during your colonic. Massage of certain Meridian points also helps stimulate detoxification during the treatment.

Your holistic colon hydro therapist will often (not always) be trained in a variety of alternative healing methods like Iridology, Acupuncture, Massage, Aromatherapy, Nutrition etc. The therapist will be able to tell you after the session which organs need more support / strengthening, if there is Candida overgrowth or parasites in your system. How well your food is digested and which foods are not digested hence better left from your diet. Most holistic colon Hydro therapists will be sensitive enough to see or feel emotional/ spiritual issues relating to your digestion and wellbeing during the session.

Colonics are best done in the morning. It is advisable to relax before and after the colonic and it is good to drink some water before and after colonics. Do not eat 2 hours before the Colonic. After the colonic, you may take a detoxification bath and/or drink a green juice (e.g. wheatgrass). The body must be free from digesting solid food to repair and detoxify. It is better to eat early so the body can repair and detoxify while sleeping. Therefore, eat at least three hours before going to bed.

The colonic procedure is not offensive, not painful, and takes approximately one hour. The cost can be between $80 and $140 in Australia. Some clinics give a discount on a series of treatments.

The purpose of a colonic procedure is to remove toxic material, relieve intestinal stress, stimulate intestinal muscle function, reconditioning of intestinal muscles and elimination. The movement should be twenty-two beats per minute to process the waste food through the colon.

With colon irrigation, your sense of wellbeing is often dramatically improved. You feel lighter and more energetic. The body can again take nourishment from food and defend itself against disease. Natural peristalsis, tone and regularity are restored and many serious diseases may be averted through this gentle, sterile, scientific technique.

If you do not have a movement for each meal you eat, then you need help to get your system in shape. The quickest improvement for those having colonics is their energy level. They are not as tired as prior to colonics. Next the skin condition is improved. Other benefits are better assimilation of nutrients, less body odour and bad breath, and less belly distention.

The importance of keeping our body clean inside as well as out cannot be over emphasized. You will not be able to secure good health unless you clean out your system and these systems can't be cleaned out if the main drain is sluggish or blocked up. Our colon is the main drain. If you could see what has come out of people's unhealthy colons, you would hardly believe it. In autopsies on colons, seventy percent of the bodies had encrusted fecal matter, worms and impaction in the colon.

If you think your colon is clean because of your bowel habit, let's consider a few more facts. Out of one hundred people, there may be one or two not having matter lining the walls and pockets of the colon. Of the other ninety-eight, there are probably fifty who have some very heavy encrustments in the colon; of the other forty-eight, about half will have up to three and a half kilos of matter lining the colon, and the other half will have up to two and a half kilos.

Colonics will not only tell you if you have parasites but also help to remove them. Some symptoms of parasites include, restless sleeping, fatigue, poor assimilation and absorption of nutrients, food cravings (especially for sugars and breads), as well as an inability to feel satisfied after a large meal.

Colonic will also help improve the beneficial bacteria in your bowel. Even though some good and bad bacteria will be washed out during the session, it is much easier for the body to reproduce beneficial bacteria after a session when bad bacteria and waste have been reduced.

If you tried it once, you know why so many people love it. The benefits outweigh any concerns that you might have. It is absolutely safe and a surprisingly pleasant procedure if done by a well-trained holistic practitioner. View www.shanti.com.au.

I used the open system and found it very comfortable, I read a book during my sessions and the practitioner came in when I called her to give me a wheat pack for my stomach, which I found helpful. It is very private and I had such amazing results.

You can find some more Information on colonics by www.shanti.com.au.

Detoxing with raw foods:

Detoxing is not always about what herb, or pill, you can take. The body detoxes daily as a normal function of the body. Raw food allows the body to perform its natural function by reducing the energy used to break down chemicals and cooked food material and is able to break it down and use it very fast and effectively.

After careful consideration and discussion with your health care professional, remember about the detoxing effects of a raw food diet. It may be possible to experience withdrawal symptoms like headaches and flu like symptoms. Especially if you delete coffee, or alcohol or some other drugs from your daily intake.

As mentioned earlier keeping a 90 to 98% raw food diet will work well for detoxing, decreasing that percentage as you move into the maintenance diet. It all depends how unwell you feel, as to how long you may decide to stay onto the high percentage raw diet.

There are many people on this diet for many years. My recommendation is to seek the advice of a health care professional such as a Naturopath, preferably registered with a governing association, such as the Australian Traditional Medicine Society in Australia. Most Naturopaths in Australia have 4 diplomas that make up their Naturopathic Diploma. They have a Diploma in Nutrition (very different to a Dietician) Diploma in Herbal Medicine, Diploma of Homeopathy and a Diploma of Remedial Therapy.

The person who inspired me to go raw was Dan MacDonald in America. You can research him on YouTube, the Life Regenerator. I highly recommend you seek him out. He has DVD's and more than a thousand inspiring messages for you to make the transition, he also interviews people who have healed themselves of all sort of illnesses.

I also find Dr Joseph Mercola and his interviews invaluable as well as Dr Eric Berg.

Detoxing language:

I have referred several times to the work of Dr Emoto where he demonstrates a change in water, when crystalizing in his experiments, regarding the water being exposed to certain words, messages, music and other experiments.

My strong intuitive view is that words, as well as thoughts, are quite powerful and therefore useful. They have an impact on strengthening the body or weakening the body.

For example, if you are constantly criticized, denigrated everyday, even though you try to protect yourself, by contradicting what is said, (even making excuses for other's behaviour) this environment is not healthy.

If we look at deleting from our everyday language, language that is not serving us, an example and only the beginning of what could be a long list is following. Everyone is an individual with their own set of words that make up their everyday language, like sayings, beliefs unconscious or conscious.

EXERCISE: LANGUAGE DELETE

Delete exercise:

I should do this or that.
Replace:
I could do this or that.
Delete:
I wish I could do this or that,
Replace:
I choose to do this or that

Take responsibility for yourself and your words, your language, your life.

DETOXING WITH EXERCISE

Assisting the body to detox naturally, using its normal function can be achieved by exercising which aids the lymphatic system to move toxins out of the body.

Some of the signs and symptoms experienced with this process and any other detoxing is odour under the arms, bad breath, profuse sweating, just to name a few. The experience is different for everyone. I believe there is a clinic in Melbourne Australia where they use exercise as well as other forms of detoxing and help to treat people with CFS.

It is important to note that people with CFS will experience negative symptoms when exercising, the time spent exercising is limited and usually beneficial when the body feels strong enough to withstand it.

Visualizing doing an exercise routine is another form of achieving these results too.

DETOXING WITH BREATHING

Taking very deep breaths will allow the lungs to pump and expel air, increasing the quantity of oxygen that you make available to your body, lymphatic system as well as cardiovascular system. I heard an interview with a man who had fallen out of a plane, much of his body crushed by the impact. He was a quadriplegic and the doctors gave him little hope of recovery. All he could control was his breath and his brain and he used this to his benefit, healing himself, finally walking. A wonderful reminder of the power of the breath.

DETOXING WITH WATER

Think about the water quality that you take every day, ask yourself, "Is it alkaline, acidic, does it have chemicals or heavy metals in it. How much do I take?" Our body is mostly water, so how much do you think we rely on it for our bodily processes? Water is the conduit for our hormones, electric impulses, and who knows what else not discovered yet. Some theories are that water has its own entity, it is alive, hearing and reacting to words for example.

There is a lake in Japan where monks go to pray, and it is said that the water quality has improved since the practice began.

DETOXIFYING WITH ZEOLITE

Zeolites are natural volcanic minerals that are mined in certain parts of the world. (Australia has mines in WA) When volcanoes erupt, molten lava and thick ash pour out. Because many volcanoes are located on an island or near an ocean, this lava and ash often flows into the sea. Thanks to a chemical reaction between the ash from the volcano and the salt from the sea amazing minerals like zeolites are formed in the hardened lava over the course of thousands of years.

EXERCISE: ZEOLITE

Wash your hands with a normal, heavily scented, perfumed, soap.

Then wash your hands again with Zeolite powder. Observe the difference.

It will take away the scent of the soap and your hands will smell clean and earthy is the only description I could give this.

(Zeolites action is to absorb chemicals) The more you wash your hands with Zeolite the more it will absorb unwanted chemicals from your body. Slow but steady process. Long term exercise.

Use Zeolite to soak your feet, as a face mask, mouth wash, under armpits, on your glands around your neck, be creative.

Have zeolite powder in small shaker bottles by the taps and wash your hands often with it and use it as a mouth wash 10 times per day at first, it will start to feel different, you may notice your breath smells better and your sore throat starts to improve.

RAW DIET CHALLENGE

HOME WORK

Some theories on the effects of the Raw Diet and its effect on the endocrine system; Dr. N. W. Walker has said that the best way to keep the hypothalamus healthy is by eating mostly raw foods. Noxious substances from improper foods can slowly destroy the hypothalamus, which is actually the body's thermostat.

He talks about toxins in the bloodstream, from poor elimination, and a poor diet which he theorizes being a struggle factor for the hypothalamus. He talks about the hypothalamus function regulating appetite and sleep patterns and its connection with the pituitary gland and the effect of regulating body temperature and this having an effect for people with immune function disturbances.

With people suffering from CFS a common denominator is the continuous sore throats and swollen glands. Dr Walker has an interest and studied glandular health and diet. He believes that if we keep the hypothalamus and pituitary glands happy with a proper diet and exercise it may have a positive effect on the immune system.

One of the first reactions, or visible changes, that occur when you start on the raw diet, from my own experience and observation, is the change in your lymphatic fluid. The viscosity and the reduction of pooling in certain areas of your body like the underarms, ankles wrists, neck, reduce, making you look thinner, but, not necessarily reflected on the scales.

There is a definite change to the actual feel of the body. Your skin starts to look and feel improved, smoother, with increased elasticity. You can test by pulling the skin on the top of your hand, (the opposite side of your palm), pinch, hold and release. You will notice the skin returns to normal quite quickly. Do these exercises on someone who is dehydrated, the skin takes a longer time to return to normal. Before I went on to the raw food diet my skin was slow to returning, with a noticeable lack of elasticity.

WEEK ONE:

In this exercise it is important to record and compare symptoms from week 1 to week 2 and forward results to my email address on my website. Please let me know if you are happy to publicize your results and whether you would like your name included in the findings. I am hoping this will help, encourage and give hope to other chronic fatigue syndrome sufferers.

MONDAY TO SUNDAY 7 DAYS

Eating as normal, doing the activities as normal.

Please note: Do not change bedrooms or environment within these two weeks. Keep taking the same drinks and medications etc.

SYMPTOM LIST

Please record your symptoms of CFS or Fibromyalgia or Chemical Sensitivities.

Example:

Restless sleep

Restless legs

Headache 1 -10 scale: 3 headaches this week at a scale of 6 out of 10 scale.

Aching muscles: score the pain (Also please note if some days were worse than others)

Aching joints: score the pain

Swollen glands in the neck

Sore throat

Infections: Description

Weakness: Score your strength

Memory, reading ability holding focus, understanding, confusion: Score

Dizziness: Score

Sensitivities: Describe and score

OTHER description and score

WEEK TWO:

MONDAY TO SUNDAY 7 DAYS

This week will consist of a change in diet only. Please do not change your medication or anything else you might be taking.

DISCLAIMER: PLEASE NOTE: This is a voluntary exercise and seeking the advice of your General Practitioner is advisable and recommended prior to engaging in this exercise.

RAW DIET

BREAKFAST: Juicing
2 very large glasses of fresh juice.

JUICE: Green apple, celery, ginger, green spinach or kale or both (handful) or 3 to 4 leaves. coriander, lime or lemon. (Every morning, this is the basis of the green juice detox) Freshly squeezed and drunk within 15 minutes of making. Add beetroot and carrots if you like.

SNACKS: bananas, dates, oranges, any fruit or any nuts or coconuts (lots of) Cashew spread, Tahini, other nut pastes to put on carrots or celery or smoothies etc.
LUNCH: Salad
Anything vegetable in the salad, no dressing, salt and pepper, oil and vinegar only. (no balsamic vinegar)
Example 1: lettuce, raw corn from the cob not the frozen stuff, capsicum, snow peas and mushrooms cut thinly.
Example 2: zucchini shredded with tomatoes and snow peas and shredded carrots.
Example 3: zucchini shredded with a topping of tomatoes, shallots garlic salt pepper and basil (in the blender) for the sauce to go on top of zucchini.
Example 4: Soup (raw) Juice carrots and put juice in blender with one avocado salt and pepper small garlic optional, or herbs like coriander (optional)

Example 5: Spinach, capsicum, and avocado with chili if you like, garlic salt pepper.
NOTE: Go on the internet for more inspiration.

DINNER: Soup, Salad, Juice (2 big glasses), or smoothie
Soup: juice 5 carrots and put half an avocado or a full one then salt and pepper.
Smoothie examples:
Almond milk and bananas
Almond milk and berries
Almond milk and cherries, apricots, figs etc.
TEAS: green teas of any kind

DELETE: Coffee and alcohol, or any other stimulants like black tea, and alcohol related products. No wheat, dairy, sugar, no processed foods of any kind. Only raw fruit vegetables seeds and nuts.

Then after two weeks rate all your previous symptoms.

Restless sleep
Restless legs
Headache 1 -10 scale: 3 headaches this week at a scale of 6
Aching muscles: score the pain (Also please note if some days were worse than others)
Aching joints: score the pain
Swollen glands in the neck
Sore throat
Infections: Description
Weakness: Score your strength
Memory, reading ability holding focus, understanding, confusion: Score

Dizziness: Score
Sensitivities: Describe and score
OTHER description and score

RETURN YOUR "Raw Diet Challenge" TO:
Karyl Sanchez
Chronic Fatigue Shop
www.chronicfatigueshop.com.au

Sensitivities experienced by a chronic fatigue sufferer reacts well with detoxing it is the best we have and no, I do not feel its futile to detox even if there will be more toxins encountered along the way. What seems to be the major effect of detoxing for the CFS sufferer is that the body seems to go through a process, like the computer hitting the reset button. Once you detox and you reset your body, you tend to deal with toxins and viruses more efficiently from then on.

NOTE: Find what gives YOUR BODY the most stressful response. This is particularly crucial, e.g. it could be amalgams, or a gold crown, or it could be an underlying infection in the gums or anywhere in the body. It could be, where you are sleeping, e.g. on ley lines. Or a chronic stressful relationship, or work situation, many other scenarios.

Once you start making changes, and you build on the successes, the spiral upwards starts becoming visible and your faith in healing becomes stronger. The bleakness of this syndrome starts to shift. Imagining life without CFS will start to become a reality.

Chapter 5

SENSITIVITIES

Chronic fatigue syndrome, Fibromyalgia, Myalgic Encephalitis, chemical sensitivities, yuppy flu, etc when these symptoms are manifesting you will become "SENSITIVE."

This is the only way I can describe what actually happens to the body, because so many systems in the body are interrupted. Unlike cancer, or heart disease, or any other illness of a specific area.

Unique to CFS sufferers sensitivity is so subtle yet profound that full attention and acknowledgement must be given or the negative aspects will overwhelm any positives that may evolve from this syndrome.

Sensitivities may be found in:

LIGHT

When you are in the stages of CFS that are acute or even long term, light sensitivity seems to be common and is an affliction that could be managed with sunglasses if you go out. Alternating cold and hot packs to the eye area and forehead. Herbal cream by Pinnacle Health

Clinic in Parramatta NSW Australia, rubbed on the sinus area of the face, the throat on the glands, under the armpits and on the souls of the feet, this cream has many benefits to list.

Massaging the muscles of the eyes yourself is beneficial if done gently and slowly. Acupresure and acupuncture treatments are also helpful. Cranial Sacral Practitioners can do some great work for people with any head and neck issues sometimes Osteopaths train in this therapy and you may find them under the Osteopathic Association. It is important to mention that when your body starts to heal that the sensitivities start to decrease.

SOUND

Any natural sound is a great enhancer of energy, like birds, water cascading, the ocean, the waves, the breeze through the trees, the frogs or crickets etc.

Sounds that you may find offensive, can play havoc with your energy supply and drain you very quickly, if you notice it, remove the offensive noise and rebalance by listening to a sound you find soothing and breathing exercises usually helps.

Its all about vibrations.

For example someone yelled at me which I found was very jarring and upsetting. The actual repercussions of that behavior lasted over 3 days the vibration was so strong that the bodies reaction was so profound. The first day I was crying and in a daze, the second I was still in a daze and felt very sensitive and drained the same as the third day but felt better than the first day. Similar to a chemical reaction but of course with the emotional component.

It is interesting to note that when a CFS sufferer is in an acute stage of the illness they usually can not tolerate much noise at all.

TASTES

Some lollies or sweets, or foods that have preservatives, or flavorings can cause an allergic reaction where the symptoms of CFS will flare up. For example, great weakness, nausea, dizziness, numbness, foggy brain great tiredness and your eyes just want to close. Foods that contain aspartame is a good one to double check and avoid. Yellow cordial drink is another. To some people red cordial drinks as well. There are so many on the market that its too hard to list. Preference is water. Slightly alkaline even better and freshly squeezed juices. Take an antihistamine, this may help.

ODOURS

Be wary of perfumes, some can cause an allergic or sensitivity reaction and can trigger an episode of CFS symptoms. In this case an antihistamine works well. The packet may say for hay-fever but it works well with an allergic reaction to smelling a perfume or smelling fresh paint, garden chemicals and fertilizer. It depends on the individual as to what triggers an allergic reaction. Its not always recognised as an allergic reaction because the reaction to a CFS sufferer is manifested by the cfs symptoms, not runny noses or skin rashes.

PAIN

The pain reactions of a chronic fatigue suffer, have baffled many doctors and physiotherapists. They experience pain and pain reactions that travel all over the body, with no particular pattern or causative reason. It seems to have a random activity pattern. Sometimes connected to emotional stress other times, allergic reactions and sensitivities in the body. My experience with pain has been as described above with an emphasis on my weaknesses in certain areas of the spine such as neck cervical. There has been some involvement of vagus nerve reactions in connection to pain responses. Mainly while being treated by the physiotherapist or osteopath on the neck area. I feel there is a connection with high pain and the vagus nerve reaction. I have not reacted when the pain is low.

Sometimes when you are feeling undue amounts of pain, it is better to calm the nervous system down before getting treatment. Deleting coffee or any other stimulant before the appointment, and drink a good amount of water. Hydration is very important before treatments when you know a vagus nerve reaction may take place.

Breathing exercises and the Amygdala training technique is very useful here.

CHEMICALS

Sensitivities to chemicals as in cleaning products, deodorizers, aromatherapy candles or plugg-ins in room deodorizers, certain food colourings for example as in yellow or red cordial, food enhancers in sauces and other packaged products, chemicals in anesthetics and medication (dentistry and surgery).

There again hydration, delete coffee or black tea, breathing technique and amygdala retraining technique as well as a handy antihistamine packet in your bag would not go astray. Remembering the natural antihistamine options.

DENTISTRY

Some research shows an improvement of symptoms with the removal and detoxing of amalgam feelings. My own experience has been of improvement with the removal of a gold crown (molar). Not a little bit but a huge and very noticeable difference in symptoms. My neck glands had reduced, lymphatic area to my wrists and hands also reduced.

I have used Zeolite powder (raw product) to detox the gold metal from my body. I wash my hands regularly with this, bath, brush my teeth, gargle, face mask, zeolite packs under my arm pits and go to sleep with these.

I have also used the muscleFX herbal cream by Pinnacle Health in Parramatta NSW Australia, the same way under arm pits.

EMF (Electromagnetic Field)

Dr Peter Dingle explains the negative effect of EMF and other under publicized electromagnetic radiation, such as computers, microwave ovens, mobile phones, radar systems and power lines, etc. There is also the issue of too much natural radiation like sun burn and its negative effects on the immune system.

Extract: Dr Peter Dingle.

"Microwaves can also be used to generate heat through the extremely rapid reversal in the polarity of electrons affected by magnetic and electric fields via a tube called a magnetron - this occurs in almost every kitchen and restaurant throughout the industrialized world, with the ubiquitous microwave oven.

Microwaves and radio-frequencies represent one of the most common and fastest growing environmental influences about which anxiety and speculation are spreading. Yet very little is known about the results of exposure to microwaves; even less is known about the relative dangers of different sources of microwaves. We do, however, know that microwaves can be reflected, transmitted or absorbed by matter in their path. Absorption occurs in matter that contains moisture, including human beings.

Living organisms absorb microwaves and radio-frequency energy at the molecular, cellular, tissue and whole body levels. Heating of internal organs is a consequence of the absorption of energy. The energy is absorbed by water within the tissue; so tissues with high water density and low blood density, such as the eyes and testes, are particularly vulnerable."

I found this information interesting and with the sensitivities of chronic fatigue syndrome sufferers, these thing can affect us easily.

PSYCHIC

There is a line of thought where CFS sufferers have been awakened psychically. Their sensitivity to their surroundings have become more acute and their abilities to "sense" has changed. Some people are more audible (clairvoyant) sense things in the form of sound, some more visual clairvoyants (clear vision) sometimes sense through dreams and visions. They see spirits or ghosts, some sensing, also called empaths, which are common. They sense through emotions and feelings (clairsentient) they just know things, some people have had their abilities to heal themselves or take to healing others.

Clairsentient is another term frequently applied to empaths. A clairsentient "just knows things" and can't always tell you how.

Precognitives sense the future in dreams or waking visions. This is usually a specific form of clairvoyance, though empaths can project forward with emotion to view a predicted outcome.

Psychometrists have the ability to sense through, feelings and to re-live events by handling personal items (jewelry or clothes) or by touching other people.

Mind readers, they are generally called telepaths, they can read mental vibrations, the way empaths use emotions, these are not so common.

Mediums read or see or sense ghosts, spirits and angelic guides.

Channels, like mediums are sensitive to spirits, but they may allow a spirit or guide temporary access to their own senses in order to facilitate direct communication. Sometimes referred to a conscious channel, which will remain in control of all their faculties during the experience and has full recollection. An unconscious channel may black out and have no recollections.

There are people who are also hyper-sensitives, who can be any kind of psychic, but the problem for them is that they cannot seem to shut off their abilities even when the information they receive is painful, overwhelming or even confusing. They tend to be empaths but may have additional abilities such as mediumship.

There are other sensitivities such as psychic smells or ghostly touches but they are secondary to the main talent such as medium etc.

If you have experienced any of these types of sensitivity, as a sole event or a regular occurrence simply know that you are now sensitive this way and embrace it. No need to analyze and "freak out" concentrate on being happy and joyful. See it as a positive experience coming from the emotion of love.

If you feel that you need to have some support in this area, visit the association for this industry in your own country and educate yourself regarding this sensitivity.

EMOTIONALLY

This has been a very interesting aspect of the illness, which is not covered or documented greatly. Generally when you are sick with a flu, for example you feel a little emotionally sensitive, and as soon as you recover you feel confident and strong again. But when you have a chronic illness like CFS, it affects you daily and long term, similar to the other symptoms of CFS. So when the symptoms are highlighted, so is the emotional sensitivity and the weak demeanor.

You become sensitive to people's comments; you may over react to comments when you would have normally not been bothered at all. The emotions felt vibrate for a longer time period than usual, your reaction to a criticism for example are deeply felt and your 'shrugging off' abilities are not strong like they used to be. There may be a strong correlation with your cognitive abilities, the brain function is just not the same as it used to be. However, once your body becomes stronger again and the symptoms of CFS become less, your reactions to emotions are much better, the feelings of being emotionally stronger are more prominent. For example if you get one of those comments of "you are not sick, you don't look sick, your faking your illness," this will no longer affect you the same way as it used to, you will no longer feel that deep hurtful emotion once felt by such comments. I am not saying that it will not cease being a nasty detrimental comment. It will always be. But, your emotional strength will return.

I have to agree with Dr Myhill's comment "where there is sensitivity, there will be toxicity, and vice versa."

Dr Sarah Myhill's book (extract)

Looking for sensitivity to chemicals

a. Lymphocyte sensitivity test for chemicals, heavy metals, silicones, VOCs. This is helpful if you suspect that you are reacting to one/some/all of those substances, in other words you are sensitive to them. I often use this where there is a silicone implant to help decide if it should be removed. Where there is sensitivity, there will be toxicity, and vice versa. Indeed, multiple chemical sensitivity is usually triggered by toxicity.

More recently John McLaren-Howard has developed similar tests to diagnose electrical sensitivity.

Information on Thyroid and pesticides (24th October 2011)

Pesticides Damage Thyroid

25 February 2010: Your thyroid gland plays an important role in regulating your metabolism and energy use. There is growing evidence linking pesticides to thyroid problems. This study examined 16 500 women living in Iowa and North Carolina who were married to men seeking certification to use restricted pesticides. They found that 12.5 per cent of the women had thyroid disease with seven per cent having underactive thyroids (hypothyroidism) and two per cent having overactive thyroids (hyperthyroidism). In the general population the rate of diagnosed thyroid disease ranges from one to eight per cent. The study found that organochlorine pesticide use was associated with a 1.2 times greater risk of hypothyroidism. Exposure to fungus killers benomyl and maneb/mancozeb doubled or tripled the chances of hypothyroidism respectively. Maneb/mancozeb also doubled the women's risk of hyperthyroidism. The herbicide paraquat almost doubled the likelihood of hypothyroidism. Yet another example of how your environment can impact your health.

Source: American Journal of Epidemiology.

My own experience with sensitivities:

In reference to sensitivities, not only my experience with the gold molar, I was also sensitive to mould (black mould) at home. My sensitivity did not allow me to use bleach, so I had someone else use bleach on the bathroom mould build up while I was away and it was kept under control with continuous cleaning using vinegar.

Soon after a gall bladder attack I went on a very strict diet to reduce the inflammation and support the liver and hopefully soften the stones. I also did a gall bladder cleanse. After my 1st cleanse I noticed that bleach was not affecting me like it used to, and my body was tolerating it now.

Of course, I don't push it, by using bleach every day, but I just do not have that terrible reaction as I used to.

I have had reactions to perfumes, especially cheap perfumes, they send me straight to sleep, my eyes close, my body becomes weak and I collapse into bed with body pain and stiffness and joint pain.

So my advice and my experience is that detoxing has definitely played a very large part in reducing the symptoms of CFS.

Another very important aspect about being sensitive and what to do to combat a reaction is to consider natural antihistamines.

The body's function when dealing with an allergic reaction is it produce histamines which react with foreign substances. So taking anti-histamines stops or reduces this natural reaction of the body. Some of these reactions are the coughing sneezing, swelling, inflammation, redness, nasal congestion and throat congestion and swelling. However, in the chronic fatigue syndrome sufferer) the brain fog, body pain, heaviness of the body), this process of the body inhibits (reduces or stops) the allergen to affect the body in a major way.

As I understand it the better the functioning of your immune system the better the body deals with allergies as well. So I guess the key is to improve your gut function, seeing a large proportion of the activity for the immune system is there and therefore you will also improve the allergic reactions.

Pharmaceutical developed antihistamines, are useful when you have a bad, uncomfortable or life threatening reaction to an allergen, for example paint. If you have had an even worse reactions, the "epi pen" is what is commonly used. This pen (epinephrine) uses and drains your supply of adrenaline to pump what is causing a reaction in your body, out, through, sweat, urine, faeces.

The adrenal gland, that sits on top of the kidneys, have our natural adrenaline stores, when they are fatigued it affects generally.

My theory is this supply from the adrenal gland is not working properly, affecting the bodies ability to detox, causing an accumulative affect, an action that has an affect on, the liver and its functions, the gall bladder and its function, the kidneys, the hypothalamus, the thymus, the amygdala. I see the endocrine system as our pump and in CFS sufferers its not working well. Just clarifying this is my own unsubstantiated theory, it is not based on any work I have read.

If you refer to the theories section of the book I explain that I feel there has been a reaction between either the quality of the epinephrine manufactured and used world wide or the body is no longer dealing effectively with the amount that we are consuming of this particular product. Possibly it is reacting to other chemicals that we intake or are exposed to everyday in our environment.

I think its also interesting noting the side effects of antihistamine medication; drowsiness, slow reaction time, and difficulty concentrating are also some CFS symptoms. These symptoms also appear after being exposed to an allergen like paint, for example, or after doing too much, or after a stress response.

If the action of antihistamines is to change, or make the body pump through natural adrenaline to get rid of the offending allergen, it could be argued that in chronic fatigue syndrome sufferers adrenal gland may be depleted or damaged and the natural adrenaline is disrupted or the pathways are disrupted. Therefore, the body does not act normally, therefore, the body is ineffective in detoxing some allergens.

NATURAL ANTIHISTAMINES

Nettle, stinging Nettle
Cardamon
Parsley
Evening Primrose
Ginger
Chamomile
Saffron
Fennel
Anise
Basil
Echinacea
Thyme

Herbs are not the only useful antihistamine, Cybele Pascal suggests 3 other useful foods. View www.cybelepascal.com and www.homeremedieshaven.com.

Foods with Vit.C e.g. lemons, guavas, blackcurrant, red capsicum, mango, kale, peaches, citrus fruits, cauliflower, spinach, kiwi fruit, bananas, honey dew melons, pineapple, cranberry juice, turnips, strawberries, black eye peas, green peas, green onions, lima beans, yellow squash, red cabbage and more.

Omega 3 fatty acids, like salmon, flax seed oil, hemp seed oil (very strong in taste and very green), walnuts, grass fed meat.

EXERCISE: SENSITIVITIES LIST

Write down a sensitivities list, give this list to your family and friends. It is more likely that they will remember and be more attentive to your sensitivities.

Here is an example:

Perfumes: cheaper style perfumes, name a few.
Deodorant sprays
Toilet Deodorisers
Plugg in Deodorisers
Cleaners, floor cleaners, bleach.
Disinfectants, with heavy perfumes.
Petrol fumes at the Petrol Stations.
Paint fumes (new or freshly painted rooms or furniture)
New carpet or rubber matts.

EXERCISE: LIPSTICK AND CHEMICALS

Using Zeolite powder, after you wash your hands with or handle heavily perfumed soap or chemical powders, to neutralize the chemicals before they are absorbed through your skin.

Soaking your feet and hands regularly with zeolite powder. You can also use bi carbonate soda to alkalinize the body, such as foot baths.

Cosmetics, can also be a form of sensitivities for some people. Check, especially the lipstick, if it has any form of lead, this would be a useful exercise to do. This technique is easy and quick, take your lipstick and place a mark with it on the back of your hand and using a gold ring preferably 14 or 18k gold, rub the ring on the lipstick mark vigorously, if the lipstick colour turns black or starts to become darker it may contain lead, the darker the mark becomes the more possible lead it contains.

EXERCISE: VISION STRESS

Another helpful hint comes from my training in Kinesiology. Placing one hand on the back of your head near your neck area and the other on your forehead, and hold for a while, this is great to balance the occipital area and frontal bone areas, for vision stress.

What you sometimes feel is that one area is more active "like electricity" than the other. You need to hold the hands there until both areas feel exactly the same. Sometimes you feel one area colder than the other or hotter.

EXERCISE: OM OR AMEN HUMMING

This exercise very useful after an allergic reaction, or when you are tired or when your brain is over active.

My suggestion is to balance the body with sound, humming correction is a kinesiology technique I practice. You take a breath in and as you breath out you hum. The words Amen are also good to use as well as OM. They will vibrate through out the body. This technique is done standing up and you do this until you feel that the vibration has gone through the whole body.

Sometimes you can experience the vibration getting stuck in certain areas, maybe the stomach or the legs or the throat. You need to continue until you feel that it is vibrating through the whole body. If a practitioner is with you when you are doing this technique she can pick up where you are being stuck. A very useful technique to master.

This technique will help to de-stress you, it will help to balance your body, it will help to calm your body and your mind, it will release any blockages and allow your body to work better. You can even feel sometimes that your lymphatic system flows better. Your breath will be deeper and stronger and it has a wonderful affect on calming the central nervous system.

EXERCISE: ODOUR REACTIONS

This is not necessarily an exercise but a product that you need to keep close at hand. It is useful if you can tolerate the pharmaceutical product of antihistamines. It does not matter if it says its for hay fever, it works well if you have a reaction to smelling paint for example or inhaling perfume or other chemicals.

I also carry "Rescue Remedy" which is a bach flower remedy for stress, and for kids who throw tantrums, but it is handy when you have suffered any form of stress reaction.

When you have a reaction such as this, it is also beneficial to go into a meditative state and use the breath to calm the system down, talk slowly, calm your energy down and stay very still, do not use any excess energy to do other things. Even eating. Spend time calming down and let your body recover from the allergic reaction that the paint fumes etc. caused your body.

HSP (highly sensitive people)

Stuff happens to you when your down. Anyone notice this? HSP, Highly Sensitive People, whether you are now or you were prior to the illness, it is now undeniably how you are. As I understand it, you process much more information about a particular situation than most, therefore when something goes wrong and you have to disconnect from that person or situation it becomes a little more difficult than how a normal person would experience that situation. I say normal person, but what is normal relative to? As I understand there is 10 to 20% of the population that fit into this HSP category. I find that substantial. So keeping your boundaries and staying authentic with yourself is important. Respect, value and finding self worth.

Sensitivity is not the opposite of strength. Some people may perceive it as that but that is their judgement, it doesn't have to be yours. Find ways in which to respect and value how being sensitive is special and valuable. Are you hanging around people who are not so emotional? Are you idealizing that behaviour because you are emotional? How can you expect a person who is less emotional than you to value a HSP? I think it would be like asking and expecting a footballer to suddenly and out of the blue start loving ballet and everything ballet. Its just not in their experienced world, they love football.

Chapter 6

HEALING

I have an intrinsic belief that the human body is very capable of self healing with the right support. I understand the role the mind-body connection has in the manifestation of dis-ease, the dis - ease state and the importance of allowing love to heal on all levels. I embrace the concept that we all have a soul. The immortal and powerful aspect of self that connects us all to source. This world view and belief fueled my determination to seek solutions.

I never lost faith that I would and could heal, and believe me, I was challenged. Many times the black pit of despair threatened to overwhelm me with fear, confusion, feelings of loneliness and being misunderstood and uncared for.

With my health at rock bottom, the imperative necessity for change was undoubtable. I learnt the value of detoxing the body, methods to calm the central nervous system and discovered ways to reduce the impact of environmental stimuli.

David R. Hawkins, MD, PhD states in his book 'Power vs Force' "We think we live by forces we control, but in fact we are governed by power from unrevealed sources, power over which we have no control." I see healing in this light. We need to have faith in our ability to heal. We don't have to understand the process.

Information and knowledge is power. As I researched and discerned the information that resonated with me personally, it set me on a path of self confidence, new beginnings and built my self awareness. This in turn made me stronger and more receptive to experience healing.

Hindu and Buddhist texts describe energy points in the non-physical or energy body as chakras. This concept has been embraced by many modern healing practices. One specific chakra, known as the solar plexus, I believe could play a role with CFS. When this chakra has very low energy or is blocked, the person may feel victimised and powerless in relation to self, other people, circumstances and things. They may have a tendency to give power away to others as a perceived necessity to keep peace in relationships. This chakra or energy area is usually connected with personal power, self-esteem, freedom from shame, self-worth, and self-image.

When this chakra or energy centre is unblocked or opened you may experience a strong sense of your own power and how to use it in healthy ways. You admire others with power and influence and choose to mirror people who are using their personal power to project light in the world.

Explaining our first tool, Love.

Life has shown me that the more you love yourself, the more you heal.

But what is love, exactly? Love is a powerful state of being. This state may be described as, feeling calm, breath is soft your body is relaxed, your thought patterns are of loving thoughts your awareness expands to the environment your in. I feel that when you are in this "space" the body has the ability to heal itself.

Love is a state of being, not doing.

The more time you spend in this state, projecting the intent of healing a particular situation or issue, the quicker that situation dissolves. The answers to questions appear, information becomes available and then the path becomes clearer.

I feel healing is unavailable when you come from a place of fear, anger, annoyance, disappointment, pure crankiness, rage, exasperation, irritability, fury, outrage (that was me), ticked off, wrath, aggravation and bad humour. This is how I originally saw myself being affected by CFS.

The work of the Hawaiian Psychologist, Dr Hew Len Ihaleakala's was the inspiration for calling my book "From CFS with Love ". I felt that CFS was no longer a curse but a blessing. When my attitude and outlook changed my ability to look for answers became much easier. By taking back 100% responsibility for my health and my life I found what I was seeking.

The more you love yourself the more you heal.

Escapism from the pain does not heal.

The pain of not being able to heal from CFS moves in every moment of your life, every aspect of your life. Has it expressed itself in different areas?

In asking to find faith in healing, first we need to accept that this 'pain is ours to heal'. Take responsibility, acceptance and use strength and conviction within your actions and thoughts. 'Feel' the power to heal.

When you start to ASK yourself - what do I need to heal? Feel confident you will hear the answers, the more self assured you are with yourself the louder and clearer the answers become.

As Dr Vitale explains, to heal someone else or to heal yourself say, "I am sorry, please forgive me, thank you, I love you ". So for example, I am sorry you are being affected by CFS please forgive me, thank you for the experience, I love you Karyl.

This is regarding the thought that we are all one, all connected, all one with earth and the universe. It's a powerful mantra that for years had me baffled finally I think now I understand it. Dr Hew Len Ihaleakala explains this idea well and as a psychologist working in Hawaii he had the chance to heal his patients with this message. Another very important message he gives us is "Peace begins with me" and "Taking 100% responsibility." I recommend you search his work for yourselves and see if this information resonates with you.

For example I have had a strong urge for several years now that I wanted to do something to help the situation in Iraq. I asked a medium once about this and what I could do to help and she said exactly the same thing "Peace begins with me."

So the more peaceful one person becomes, that person will affect others, who will affect others and so it continues. So it's our responsibility to become more peaceful so we can eventually create an effect on the world as a whole.

As you heal yourself you will impact other parts of your life. Your family, friends and acquaintances will feel the change as your vibration expands. This ultimately has a vibrational effect on the world. As I understand, this is how it affects Iraq.

As you continue to heal you will continue to show gratitude therefore thanking yourself for believing in yourself and being open to heal from CFS. We all play a part globally in a gratitude movement.

Following is a set of exercises for healing.

BREATH

STRETCH

WALK

AFFIRMATIONS

Breathing: Take a few deep breaths. It helps to bring your awareness where it should be. As you breathe you become more conscious of "you," your body and being in the now. You may like to take a look at the work by Eckhart Tolle the Power of Now.

Relax deeply and concentrate on achieving the feeling of becoming lighter.

I found it helpful to set a reminder on my phone that at 11am every day it reminds me to take some deep breaths.

Stretch: Release any tension, restrictions as it allows your body to flow better, opening channels that may have been a bit blocked.

Yoga stretching is my favourite form of stretching as it not only works the muscles, tendons and ligaments but it also works on the meridian system and the organs associated with each yoga pose.

Walk: Walking is our pump, it allows our heart to flow, our lymphatic system to pump the white cells around the body to flow and these white blood cells clean up the lymph system of dead cells, bacteria and other such functions, Walking can warm us up, physically and emotionally. Plus it connects us with our environment, people, things, circumstances and situation. Appreciate what walking can do.

If you are too ill to walk, that's ok, visualize walking. When visualizing you can go anywhere - the beach, the country even another country, the desert or a mountain, underwater. Visualize the air, the smells, the sounds, the little creatures, butterflies, the breeze. Be as specific as you can put as much detail as possible. There are studies that have now confirmed, that when you visualize walking you are still receiving the benefit as if you are actually physically engaged in the activity.

Affirmations: Use affirmations to pave your road, the way you want it: for example, I feel calm, my day is going fantastically, everything I need is within my reach, I am so happy today, I feel light and flowing, what a beautiful day.

PAIN

Now is the time to start working on your body. Ask how do I feel, what emotion comes up for what area.

How do I feel? Example:

Fat, swollen, sensitive, stiff, aching, abandoned, lonely, scared, sensitive, vulnerable, overwhelmed, swamped?

Choose an emotion: Overwhelmed

What part of your body do you feel mostly overwhelmed? Example: heart and right shoulder.

Keep in mind, love is all that matters.

Remember when you are feeling love you cannot feel fear, and vice versa.

Ask the Divine to help you (some people ask God, some angels, some passed loved ones, some Buddha, Krishna, Mother Mary, Saints, etc) Whatever is your idea of divine is absolutely fine.

Visualise using the colour orange to heal. Take that colour and place it where the area you felt was important to heal. E.g. heart and right shoulder, then ask the Divine to help you release heavy burdens. Start to visualise a more lighter and balanced life.

You may say an affirmation, such as - harmony and clarity is everywhere.

I no longer carry heavy burdens. My life is lighter and say the word "clear" with strength and determination using a strong voice.

My health is my responsibility.

I appreciate my sensitivity by taking care of myself and focusing on my wants and needs always.

I enjoy every part of my life.

Ask the Divine please shine your light on issues that cause me confusion, conflict or worry so they may dissolve.

I view my worries acknowledge and surrender them to the light of love.

I am focused and clear on my life's direction, I know exactly what decisions to take and the opportunities I need to allow and embrace.

I make clear decisions while keeping a firm focus on loving myself.

You may have issues with other people for example, while you are dealing with these issues, make it a "big deal" to concentrate on yourself, listening carefully to yourself, helping yourself to understand, forgiving and thanking yourself as you heal yourself.

This may sound way too simple, I know, it is. How much of this have you been doing? Put a percentage 10%, 20% or 5%.

Concentrate on healing yourself and as you do, a wonderful side effect will become apparent. Your surrounding situations, sometimes, also heals. You start seeing difficult people or situations or circumstances slowly ease off, change or simply don't have the charge (positive or negative)(oomph, power, strength) that they once had.

AFFIRMATION

I feel light as if I am floating, my body feels strong and healthy.

It is very important when doing affirmations, that you do it with a physical smile (even if you do not feel like smiling) Positive hormones are still released when you smile.

- I feel happy.
- I am achieving and doing exactly what is perfect for me right now.
- My life is perfect just as it is.
- Thank you … . (God, higher power, universe, creator, the identity or the energy that you would say something like this to) for my beautiful body. It is perfect in every way and I love every bit of my body just the way it is.
- I have abundant courage.
- I have abundant energy and everything is well in my life.
- My family love and support me every day.

HEALING "IT'S ALL ABOUT BALANCE"

In this section we will be talking about several techniques that we can use to find balance.

- Positive Affirmations
- Smile
- Laughing
- Automatic writing
- Automatic sound (a,e,i,o,u,)
- Colour healing

- Chakra healing
- EFT – Emotional Freedom Therapy

EXERCISE:POSITIVE AFFIRMATIONS

I feel strong.

I feel happy.

I am moving around more and more every day.

My body feels relaxed.

My body feels flexible.

Let's look at what could be happening right now, an example could be:

I have a headache and my body is aching in the middle of my back my body feels heavy and tired.

What we need to do with this, is transform it into a positive affirmation. So ask yourself questions such as, if I did not have a headache and my body was not aching, how would my body be feeling?

A possible answer could be: I would feel light and free. Flowing and smooth movements would be easy and fun. I would feel strong and confident. I would be laughing and joking around.

The second part of the negative thought was that the body felt heavy and tired, so what would be the opposite of feeling this way, for you?

The answer could be: I feel strong and energetic.

EXERCISE: SMILE

A physical smile (even if you do not feel like smiling) Fake is ok, it still has the ability to releases those positive hormones.

Program your phone to a chime or some sort of reminder to smile 5 times per day. You can also add to it "breathe."

Put notes for yourself all over the house "smile" "breathe," in the toilet, the washbasin, the shower, on your shoe rack, on your mirror.

This is so important to put into place as it develops a new program in your body. You are telling your body this is how you would like your body to function from now on. It will be replacing your body's stuck program, pain program, shallow breathing program, that it's been stuck in for a while.

EXERCISE: LAUGHING

Just start to laugh, if it feels fake, do it anyway, hire some DVDs that you find funny, (comedians are today's healers). Allow yourself to laugh, do this often, every day if possible. (This is a crucial exercise.) Please note it is very important to increase your endorphins, raise cortisol and repair lung function. You need to move when you laugh, sit up in bed or even stand up when possible while laughing.

I cannot stress how important this daily habit of laughing is for a person with CFS.

You can learn more at healing laughter.org.

EXERCISE: AUTOMATIC WRITING

Automatic writing is a technique that is useful to remove your frustrations out of your head and put them onto paper. This action removes stress and allows the brain to engage in an activity involving the motor neuron skills. This then helps the stress to dissipate from going around and around in your head.

You start by thinking about the most stressful word that comes up for you at that point in time. Then without looking at the page you start writing down words, they don't have to make sense and there is no checking over the work to see if you wrote it down correctly. It does not even have to be legible, it is for your eyes only.

You can also swear or use language you would not normally use. You can write things you would not like anyone to know or write down your very deep stressful feelings.

Once you feel that you finished, pay attention to your body, scan how you feel from the top of your head to the bottom of your feet. Usually you will feel a difference from when you started. There will be a noticeable difference when you remember the stress level you began with and the stress level you feel when you finish this exercise.

Important: Burn the paper.

No one needs to see it again, not even you.

EXERCISE: AUTOMATIC SOUND (a,e,i,o,u,)

Raising your vibration with sound, this technique is used to release blockages from your body by using sound.

You need to stand up, making yourself relaxed and comfortable slightly bending at the knees. So knees unlocked.

Breathe. Count breath in for 2, hold for 2 and release for 2, make it flow.

Say "a" the sound of the vowel "a." Take a breath in and as you breathe out sound out the letter "a," while you say the sound notice how it vibrates in your body, doing this several times you will notice that it may be stuck or the body may not vibrate as well in certain areas of your body.

So the idea is to keep doing the sound until your whole body is vibrating and the sound is strong and smooth and has a good vibration throughout the whole body. Continue with the rest of the vowels, a, e, i, o, u.

EXERCISE: COLOUR HEALING

Colour healing is also a vibrational technique used in healing and changing the vibration of the body affecting the central nervous system.

Think of the colour red and give it a direction by visualising it as a detoxifying force, a blood cleanser, heat, vitality, energetic healing, a heal-ant of wounds and facilitator of adrenaline, releasing stuckness and blockages.

Light, sound, colour, magnets, electricity, radio waves etc, vibrate at different rates and are classified and used accordingly. So colour has its own measurable vibration or energy like x-rays, radio, TV or microwaves.

This energy or vibration moves and intertwines itself through and around the body. It affects the seven nerve centers of the body also called chakras, these correspond to the body's endocrine system, (the glands function is to excrete, read and maneuver hormones throughout the body).

These hormones then affect our different states of bodily functions and consciousness and personality. Each colour passing through the different chakras has definite qualities and attributes. So looking at an area that is dis-eased, it is the disharmony of vibration or energy bringing the imbalance to the glandular functions and/or in the functioning of the mind.

So this is how it is believed that meditation, positive affirmation and colour therapy can produce a change in vibration and reprogramming or re-aligning or balance via the subconscious and conscious minds.

Healing with colour by Inna Segal and her other book called the secret language of the body is quite helpful.

A colour measuring program and machine costs US$2750, it measures the vibrational scale and graphs the colour for data collection, view www.stellarnet.us. This machine could show the changes visually of your vibrational energy changes.

EXERCISE: CHAKRA HEALING

Each of the seven chakras has a corresponding colour. If you can visualise each chakra and its corresponding colour, you scan your body from top to bottom.

As you do this on an almost meditative state you may notice you have trouble visualising a particular colour for a particular chakra or the colour you visualise can't seem to spread and grow around that chakra area.

It is important then to spend time with this area or chakra and think about what the chakra governs. Which emotions or feeling does this chakra represent and what can you do to make this chakra stronger and more vibrant.

For example the root chakra is governed by the colour red. if the colour does not seem to be bright strong and radiating or maybe you just cannot visualise the red at all.

This chakra has been associated with self acceptance and wants, the body areas, hypothalamus, thalamus back of the brain, adrenals, kidneys bladder, appendix, and large intestine.

Explore what this chakra represents. Have a look at what practical things you can do to help this chakra be more vibrant.

The root chakra is also referred to as the base chakra because it is located at the bottom of the spine. The root chakra is about root support, the root of the tree supports and feeds the tree, the root chakra of the human supports and feeds and nurtures the body.

It is also connected to physical vitality and grounding. Security, the feeling and the sense of security and its relation to abundance, material security, financial power or security. As well as the sense of being possessed or about possessions either material possessions or personal possessions. Not feeling that your desires and decisions in life are being supported by others or self or circumstances or situations. For example not being able to provide for yourself, your family, threatened, fear, not belonging, and living in an unsupported world.

What can you do to make this chakra stronger? How can you make yourself feel secure and safe in this world, this environment or within your family and ultimately within yourself? How can you be more loyal to yourself? How can you assert your desires and have courage and therefore strength? Once you find how to actively do practical things to make yourself feel this way, it will manifest. As a result you will then be able to see red easily and clearly.

I had trouble with this chakra and bought myself a pair of red sunglasses which I use when I am feeling vulnerable. When I am sick and not well or just feeling weak.

An example: if you are having problems thinking, or memory problems, you have a foggy brain and you are in a sea of indecisiveness, you feel sorry for yourself, you feel insecure and you feel that you have no money for example.

What ACTIONS will you take to make this change for yourself?

Have a go at working out which chakras these feelings belong to and what affirmation you can put together for it.

HELP WITH YOUR CROWN CHAKRA

By www.inner-truth.net

Relative Questions.
If you feel an imbalance in your crown chakra. Look at the following questions honestly, to help seek balance.
It is useful to answer all the questions initially with YES / NO / MAYBE and then go back and work through all the YES answers and the MAYBE answers.
Those of you who answer YES to; can try to find a way to resolve the issue. When the issue is resolved, your ache or illness may subside.

Are you having trouble accepting something?
Are you acting/have you been acting selfishly?
Are you/have you been feeling superior?
Are your judgements based on facts?
Are you hoping for a different outcome to something?
Are you feeling alienated?
Are you feeling let down with 'life' / unsatisfied? (with the CFS illness)
Are you having trouble knowing what to do with yourself? (feeling confused)
Do you feel a lack of enthusiasm to live your life?

RE-BALANCING CHARKAS

Individual rebalancing will depend entirely on the specific issue. But it is especially good to write things down.

Please note that an imbalance is not only caused by a weakened chakra. The aim is to have all chakras in complete balance with each other. And it does not mean that we are always out of balance. Understanding that when we are out of balance it is our body's way of telling us that we need to look out for ourselves right now.

Your imbalanced body is trying to tell you some important truth about you as a person. If the score of six represents weak and the score of one represents strong, it could mean you are OVER accepting, OVER trusting, OVER creative etc. thus re-balancing must either involve increasing the size of all the other chakras or reducing the influence of the strong chakra. A good healer, who works with chakras is the best person to work with.

You may also find a Kinesiologist can help with chakras and generally balancing the energy of the body.

EFT – EMOTIONAL FREEDOM TECHNIQUE

When I first experienced EFT, I went through the motions, the tapping the affirmations but it was not until I started questioning how I FELT after I did the technique, that I started noticing the changes. So if there are changes you would like to make, this technique makes movements, shifts in the mind and body, so I use it frequently and easily now. More information is found on youtube search EFT for CFS specifically. You will also find Psychologist and Counselors use this technique as well as Kinesiologist.

EXERCISE: BALANCING WITH EFT

I like visualising the infinity sign while saying and tapping the meridian points:

Even though I ...example: have pain all over my body

I deeply love and respect myself

Even though I ...

I am alone and have to do it myself,

I deeply love and respect myself.

OR you can say I deeply love and accept myself.

Visit www.eft-universe.com, www.eft.mercola.com or www.123eft.com

WHO AM I WHEN I VALUE ME MORE? A beautiful healer from Queensland Sunshine Coast Australia, Dianne Graham said to me. This is a lovely question you can ask yourself to open up more positive aspects of looking at yourself.

I hope that sharing my journey with you is opening doors to your own path of healing.

Chapter 7

STRESS

Where are you losing energy? This is an important question to ask when you are investigating stress.

IMPORTANT NOTE: Any stressful situation will exacerbate your symptoms, no matter what stage of the illness you are at.

Reduce stress and the immune system will strengthen. With CFS sufferers it's the most single important and urgent thing to pursue.

Coffee and/or other stimulants such as drugs and excessive alcohol have an impact on CFS symptoms. It has a bearing on your adrenal glands adrenaline release. The KEY to healing from symptoms of CFS is to preserve your adrenaline.

WHAT IS STRESS?

Stress has been defined as the body's automatic physiological reaction to circumstances that require the body to have a behavioural change.

The autonomic nervous system, the limbic system (the feeling and reacting brain) performs a reaction called these days the fight or flight response or reflex. The body experiences a threat or a perceived threat, this can be physical or emotional. Whether it's in the physical form or an imagined thought, the hypothalamus gland located in the centre of the brain, causes the sympathetic nervous system to release epinephrine and norepinephrine (also known as adrenaline and noradrenaline) as well as other hormones.

When these hormones are released they activate the arousal mechanism in the body and this is viewed by noting the metabolism rate changes. Plus the heart rate, blood pressure, breathing and muscle tension all increase.

The basic understanding of the central nervous system and its connection to the endocrine system, which by my theory is not functioning at its best ability in the chronic fatigue syndrome sufferers.

It will be useful to embrace the need for stress control, one of the most important functions of the hypothalamus is to view a link between the nervous system to the endocrine system via the pituitary gland.

The hypothalamus is responsible for certain metabolic processes and other activities of the autonomic nervous system. It synthesizes and secretes certain neuro-hormones, often called hypothalamic-releasing hormones, and these in turn stimulate or inhibit the secretion of pituitary hormones. The hypothalamus controls body temperature, hunger, thirst, fatigue, sleep, and circadian cycles. So as you engage in stress there is a chemical and physiological reaction in the body.

Here are a few areas where you may like to start investigating where you may be losing energy.

Physical:

The physical body. What allergies do you have? What sensitivities do you have? When you are very sick with an overload of symptoms this task is somewhat difficult because your body is reacting to much of your environmental stimuli. So you need to spend time calming down, meditating and doing the Gupta amygdala retraining program, as well as breathing exercises (refer to the Healing chapter).

Allergies, Intolerances and Sensitivities:

These could be foods, food additives, colourings, food combinations, things that are hard to digest, medication, drugs, amalgams or gold dental molars. Think carefully about what is ingested and it's not all food. Another example, aluminium pots, cooking or eating out of a glaze bowl that may have cadmium, touching petrol or inhaling the fumes when you fill up your car at the service station, vaccines, flu shots, medication and other products.

Emotional:

Relationships, people that trigger your emotional response, passive aggressive or aggressive behaviour, work or work related issues.

ENVIRONMENTAL

Lets explore your immediate environment. This includes your house, your place of work, your shopping area, where you live, where your food and water comes from. When you start noticing symptoms, you may like to check from time to time, your environment check for mould or spores. Also consider the cleaning products used in your home or work, basically anything that you are exposed to everyday. These could be disinfectants, bench sprays, perfumes, plug ins, make up, face creams, hand creams, toothpaste.

Use only simple products and not all marked "natural" are natural. My suggestion is to see an expert such as a naturopath and get a list from them on what products are suitable for sensitive people. For example toothpaste may include sulphur derivatives and your body could be highly sensitive to this so it's reacting every time you use your toothpaste.

Unless you start finding these things out, your body will continue to have to battle with the multitudes of chemicals you are exposing yourself to and this weakens the body instead of strengthening it.

EMOTIONAL

The emotional investigations are very tricky because it could be conscious or subconscious. I find that with the help of a good Kinesiologist who can muscle test you can detect what emotions are draining you. You will find this technique a reliable and a quick therapy tool to discover where you are losing energy. Sometimes it's right in front of you and you don't see it or do not want to see it. It could bring up many issues for you and it could mean you need to change something that you know needs changing but have not wanted to deal with.

In this category you need to explore your relationships and how your body is reacting to them.

This is where healing from CFS requires your courage. You actually need to be ready to let go of things that are not working in your life.

It is very difficult, painful and scary. It is like going into battle and the battle is actually you saving your body and your soul.

Serious stuff. But do you want to heal or do you want to continue where you are right now?

If you make the latter choice be sure that you understand it is your choice and it will always be your choice.

When you look back at what you have achieved your feelings of being proud are overwhelming. There is nothing that compares. Your journey, your courage, your choice.

PSYCHICALLY

This is an interesting subject, but maybe not for everyone. If you have determination and a desire to investigate all matters relating to yourself you need to see that we are not only a physical being but also an emotional being and an energetic being. A being with actions and reactions to an esoteric world experienced by your psychic senses I explain this in the Sensitivities Chapter as well as understanding your Energy Keys in the Energy Chapter.

STRESS AND YOU

Speaking from experience when I am stressed out by a certain person or situation or incident, it is very easy for me to go into a CFS day which coincides with some virus that is floating around.

As a result the defenses lower and instead of getting the usual symptoms of the virus I get the CFS symptoms. My eyes close, I get a headache and my body aches terribly. My mind becomes foggy and cognitive speech and function are slow and slurred.

When my symptoms were very bad at the beginning of my illness, I also had swelling of the tongue. I was better by laying in bed without a pillow the straighter the body and the more time I rested, the better it was. The brain would continue to go on hyper mode and kept thinking thoughts as if it was stuck on a very active high gear.

Fearfulness of some sort, not so much of the physical but the actual mental, or psychological. I would get upset easily and could not rationalise the off the cuff comment that had been said. It may not have been a huge deal but I could not turn off the stress I felt about the incident.

It was very frustrating especially when I did not even have the energy to talk or communicate with anyone about it. I was starved for understanding and I could not explain what was happening to me.

I first experienced some sort of fog lifting experience when I stopped eating bread and sugar for 3 months. I could not believe food could do this. I explain this in detail in the My Story chapter.

The stress and fog brain symptoms were also majorly relieved by colonics and the Gupta Amygdala retraining program.

I feel the combination was the key to the results.

Detox plus Stress Relief (Gupta Amygdala Retraining) Plus Colonics plus the herbs and raw food = No C.F.S symptoms.

The stress relief not only incorporates the stress management techniques but also the removal of stress from the physical, mental, environmental, the geopathic stress lines, relationships and chemicals. So it's not only what you take out but what you bring in as well.

STRESS AND THE GUPTA AMYGDALA RETRAINING PROGRAM

This program was developed by Ashok Gupta in the UK.

The amygdala is an important structure located in the anterior temporal lobe. The amygdala makes reciprocal connections with many brain regions including the thalamus, hypothalamus, septal nuclei, orbital frontal cortex, cingulate gyrus, hippocampus, parahippocampal gyrus and brain stem. The olfactory bulb is the only area that makes input to the amygdala and does not receive reciprocal projections from the amygdala.

The amygdala is a critical center for coordinating behavioral, autonomic and endocrine responses to environmental stimuli especially those with emotional content.

It is important to the coordinated responses to stress and integrates many behavioral reactions involved in the survival of the individual or of the species, particularly to stress and anxiety.

Lesions of the amygdala reduce responses to stress, particularly conditioned emotional responses. Stimulation of the amygdala produces behavioral arousal and can produce directed rage reactions.

Various stimuli produce responses mediated by the amygdala. The convergence of inputs is important since it allows the generation of learned emotional responses to a variety of situations. The amygdala responds to a variety of emotional stimuli, but mostly those related to fear and anxiety. view www.dartmouth.edu/~rswenson/NeuroSci/chapter_9.html. www.guptaprogramme.com.

ANTI STRESS EXERCISES

SMILE:

This exercise is also explained under the Healing chapter, so engage in a smile no less than 5 times per day, even if you don't feel like it. Set the phone alarm to chime 5 times per day and take this exercise very seriously.

When smiling you activate certain muscles and body responses giving hormonal releases that send a message to our brain to reduce stress.

LAUGH:

This exercise is explained under the Healing chapter also and it is a very important exercise to be taken seriously. This again releases essential hormones to reduce stress and balance the autonomic nervous system. Watching a TV show or comedians that make you laugh needs to be part of your weekly schedule. I would also deleted watching the news or negative filled TV programs while you are concentrating on healing.

When doing Kinesiology balances this correction sometimes comes up. Once performed the body balances out and you can test the chakras or simply muscle test the body and it corrects the weakness. Kinesiology treatments are explained under the Chapter of Therapies, Products and other Techniques.

STRESS TEST

You may find it helpful taking a stress test; I have found a free stress test on the internet on www.stresstest.com which may help you to give you a start on checking your overall stress situation.

STRESS RELIEF

Taking stress out of your day is simple:

Make a commitment to yourself that taking stress out of your life is simple and necessary.

The percentage rule: If you look at your day in a percentage scale, and view that for say 20% of the day you engage in stressful activities, such as worry, yelling, negative self talk, projecting, accuse, abuse, thoughts of the past, indulge yourself in feelings of anger and much more. Do you get the idea? Then when you start filling your day with the exercises that we have spoken about in this book such as, smiling (5 times per day), watching a funny comedian minimum of once per week, taking opportunities to laugh (even if they feel false) positive affirmations morning and night, breathing exercises, Gupta amygdala retraining Programme exercises, and the change your language exercises from the Chapter Healing. Mantra affirmations (e.g.: thank you for my healing, all is well, I love you … your name …) many times during the day. This will take up that percentage of negative action you used to indulge in and you may find that there will not be enough room in the day for the negative thoughts and activities.

So there lies the new pattern which will produce change.

Having a look at negative relationships in your life present, past, and even future, like projecting what or how someone is going to be like in the future, their reactions actions and so on.

Sometimes we do not notice that they are negative relationships until you have a break from them and realize that you are feeling calm relaxed and happy, (usually you notice this in the morning when you wake up feeling happy) simply because it is the natural bodies balance to go to that state when you are not bombarded by the negative relationship.

It takes a lot of courage and support for yourself to change these relationships and also understanding, because when you no longer accept the bombardment from the negative relationship, they will not be happy with YOU. It will generate repercussions and that's when you need to have the courage to say "I love you to yourself" concentrate only on "love" and allow the adjustment to take place. Releasing the co-dependency, if you come from a place of "how can I love myself more?" as Louise Hay explains, you will notice that continuing to be bombarded by the negative relationship is certainly "not" loving yourself more.

Stress and homeopathic treatments and herbal medicine is practical, non addictive, therapies and products that we have available. Something simple like Rescue Remedy, which is a Bach flower remedy, available in any Chemist/Pharmacy, is used not only for stress and for babies having tantrums but also for allergy reactions, any body stress reactions really.

Music: how simple and beautiful is this form of therapy. It can calm us down, it can uplift us, it can excite us, and it can take you into many different types of emotional states.

Hypnosis: I have now personally used hypnosis to relieve stress and believe it is very effective. I used the Gupta Amygdala Retraining programme as well, there are CDs available with hypnotic music and sound to assist in the relief of stress. A quick reminder, reduce stress and your immune system will strengthen.

Drink water, stress dehydrates you. If you are following the plan and have started to incorporate the raw diet, you will notice that dehydration is much better now. Complete the holding of your skin test on the back of your hand to see how hydrated you are more details on this in the Detox Chapter.

It has been found that drinking coffee, black tea and other stimulants reduces the hydration in your body. So if you have one cup of coffee you may like to replace the hydration levels by drinking 3 cups of water. So if you need 1 to 2 litres of water per day, you need to make an allowance for adding more water if you drink coffee. This is something your naturopath can talk to you about. Coffee and/or other stimulants such as drugs and alcohol have an impact on stress levels. It has a bearing on your adrenal glands adrenaline release. The key to healing from symptoms of CFS is to preserve your adrenaline.

Sleep: Ashok Gupta explain that the amygdala is partly responsible for keeping people awake at night due to unconscious stress. People who have trouble with sleep engage in worrying, even though they are quite tired. The mind is bombarded with stimulated thoughts and creating a perceived danger that is unresolved so they find it difficult to get to sleep and stay as sleep. Ashok also points out that studies have shown that interrupted sleep causes further aches and fatigue the next day. So you can see how a continuous lack of sleep can accumulate and cause pain. This interrupted sleep also has an effect on the thymus and the body clock, the temperature rhythms and melatonin secretion.

The pineal gland is believed to be the regulator of sleep, this gland changes serotonin into melatonin. Melatonin is stored by the pineal gland sometimes this gland is referred to as the third eye. The gland also responds to light and dark, so the melatonin secretion slows down when the sun comes up and you are surrounded by light.

EXERCISE: LIGHT ON THE PINEAL GLAND

This exercise is generally used for people like nurses on nightshift, who may suffer from irregular sleep or interrupted sleep due to too much light and find it hard to go to sleep.

It's simple. You need a minimum of 10 minutes of sun on your face morning and afternoon. If there is no sun for a few days you can use a flashlight on your forehead between your eyebrows.

It might be an idea to incorporate this exercise with your meditation schedule as well as your smiling technique.

EXERCISE: CLEARING

Clearing not only means to cleanse or take out or remove or make clean, it also means to clear your mind of clutter and of unwanted things.

The only way to do this and stay loyal to yourself and your needs is by sorting out your wants.

Let's explain this concept. I could tell you how to do something but I will be coming from my own needs and wants. They are not your individual needs and wants so the outcome will not be tailor made for you.

What this means is that unless you are driving your own healing needs we are not going where YOU want to go. We will in fact be going where I want to go. And that is ok to start with. There is much guidance in this book but sooner or later you need to take the wheel.

Making a list of goals, acknowledging, understanding and listing your needs and your wants will ground you and give you a good steady and visible guide as well as easy reference that you can refer to in coming months.

EXERCISE: GOALS

MY goal is:
My goal for my health is:
My goal for my social life is:
My goal in relation to that particular situation/relationship/issue is:
My work/career goals are:
My financial/material issue goal is:
My spiritual goal is:

Once you have written down your goals, meditate and see how you feel. Do you feel calmer, more relaxed, and slightly stronger or is there even a definite tangible feeling of strength?

EXERCISE: MEDITATION

What is meditation? It means sit there and do nothing. Oh, it sounds so easy. But I am not sure if it is so easy if you have the symptoms of CFS. Your brain is overactive, your mind is thinking about all the pain you are feeling all over your body, while you are feeling confused and cannot focus. You might like to add, you feel like you are on a high speed merry-go-round with no stop button.

These symptoms are terrible and they do not come and go. Unfortunately they are with us all the time. That's why some doctors think that CFS is a mental disease. Remember if you come across those doctors send them "love" they are confused and need love.

Have a good laugh, remember its one of your exercises. So meditation is just like any other exercise, the more you do it the better you get at it.

Find a local meditation class and make a booking to attend this week. This is not classified under a nice thing to do; it is a MUST thing to do. No ifs and no buts.

HOW TO HANDLE A MASSIVE STRESS

Generally, people do not understand how stress affects a person with CFS or FM, they have no idea how damaging it is to these individuals. In fact, many people because they can get over stress fairly quickly cannot put themselves into the shoes of a CFS or FM sufferer.

This lack of empathy could make the stress of the stressed out CFS person escalate.

The bodies repair mechanism after stress is poor and damaged.

I believe that in these situations we do have psychologists available who are trained to deal with peek stress circumstances or post traumatic stress situations.

Forming an attitude or putting the situation into perspective and remembering that it will pass are very useful.

Seek people who support you. Do not engage with people who have shown themselves to be careless, selfish, and self-absorbed, as it will make matters worse. I can speak from experience here. Even after I have healed most of my symptoms, I am still susceptible to not recuperating fast enough from an emotional upheaval.

Usually these are times of reflection and meditation. It is very important. Breathing exercises are invaluable. Walk away from the stress if you can.

There are a number of stress reducing herbs available.

- Valerian and passionfruit flower for times of stress, this mix is usually available through your naturopath.
- There are some chemists and pharmacies that stock a mix of these herbs as tinctures; I am not as fond of the tablet forms as I feel they are not as effective as the liquid herb.
- As well as the "Rescue Remedy" a product which you can buy at a chemist or pharmacy.

Hydration is so important here, because in high times of stress the body dehydrates fast. The nerve neurons conductivity is much better when the body is well hydrated.

A massage, or a reiki session is invaluable in these situations.

Stress also makes the body acidic so several glasses of lemon juice in water would not go astray. There is on the market an Alkaliniser powder you can purchase at the health food shops.

Soaking your feet with warm water and bicarb soda will also help with alkalinity.

Remember Zinc, this is such an under rated mineral when it comes to coping with stress, immune problems and depression. Liquid Zinc.

FORGIVENESS

David Wilcock talks about the Law of One series were he explains the importance of forgiveness and service to others.

Stay integrated by forgiving yourself and others as well as things and circumstances.

Breaking through the denial is a very important step for our healing on a collective level. Taking 100% responsibility.

One of the things that happens when we are faced with a big challenge like an illness such as Chronic Fatigue Syndrome or Fibromyalgia, is that we go in circles thinking "how bad it is," but what we could do is this:

Question YOURSELF.

Questioning for Stress relief. Dr Dain Heer talks about questioning yourself to produce openness to your world of possibilities.

One of Dr Dain Heer favourite questions:

Whats right about me that I am not getting?

How can it get better than this?

In bad and good situations.

This question I love so much because it expands the mind to allow it to run wild in finding alternatives and answers to the situations at hand, in all sorts of ways.

You automatically start seeing things differently with wonder and freshness, intrigue, curiosity, love, and grace.

Just perfectly, taking you into a fantastic energy of higher love, a higher state of being, a higher vibration.

The more joy you are willing to be in, the more you will affect the world around you, as you move around, walk around, travel and connect with others.

Judging can put the breaks on your path. Clearing, asking your own energy to go back to the place where things began or were created, all the judgments, all the rejections etc, like you cant do it, etc. Let it undo. Go back and clear it.

Zero zone. Maybe this message is what Dr Hew Len was talking about as well.

Also check your feelings, is it your energy or your thoughts? WHO Does it belong to? Return it to sender. If it is not yours.

When you become sensitive, such as many people with CFS are, the confusion of being quite sensitive is very real.

As you can now appreciate, the intrinsic ins and outs of how stress can affect a person with CFS or FM. You may now begin to see how important it is to reduce it.

Chapter 8

IMMUNE SYSTEM

Trying to describe our immune system takes a large amount of background information, I will endeavor to simplify it.

The purpose of our immune system is to keep infectious micro organisms; bacteria, viruses, and fungi out of the body, and to help us fight any that have invaded the body.

The organs involved with the immune system are called the lymphoid organs. For example the adenoids, bone marrow, lymph nodes, lymphatic vessels, spleen, the thymus, the tonsils and the appendix.

The Endocrine system.

Our body's chemical messenger, utilizes hormones and the glands. Even though different hormones are found in the bloodstream these hormones affect only the cells that are genetically programmed to receive and respond to its messages. Hormone levels can be influenced by stress, infection and changes in the balance of fluid and minerals in the blood.

The endocrine system regulates mood, tissue function, growth and development as well as metabolism and sexual and reproductive process. The endocrine glands are the body's main hormone producers but other organs such as the brain, heart, lungs, kidneys, liver, skin, thymus, and even the placenta can also produce and release hormones.

The Hypothalamus is the main link between the endocrine system and the central nervous system. Nerve cells in the hypothalamus control the pituitary gland by producing chemicals that either stimulate or suppress hormone secretion.

The Adrenal glands, where the cortex produces hormones that influence stress, metabolism, the immune system and sexual development and function, the inside, called the Medulla produces (natural) epinephrine. This is also called Adrenaline. It works on increasing blood pressure and heart rate when the body needs it, when it is under stress. That is why Epinephrine (synthetic) injections are often used to counteract a severe allergic reaction.

The immune system is often much more than people assume.

Strengthen your immune system in multiple ways:

- liver detoxing
- general detoxing
- drinking water
- environmental awareness
- stress reduction
- sleeping
- addressing sensitivities

- eating raw foods
- repairing gut function

LIVER

Your liver is one of your most significant organ and detoxing your liver will be a challenging experience, but, an important one.

Learning the different functions of the liver can assist you to understand the importance of cleansing your body. The liver is supported by other organs such as the kidneys and adrenal glands.

Following is some practical information which may benefit the immune system.

CHECK LIST

1. Liver detox
2. Eating raw foods - this supports the liver by easing digestion and alkalizing the blood.
3. Releasing foods that are harmful for the liver. Alcohol, excess coffee to name a few.
4. Hot and cold packs when liver is inflamed for example using a cold pack 2 min, hot pack 10 min for about 20 minutes alternating.
5. Drinking tea that supports the liver such as green tea, dandelion tea.
6. Massaging and/or "running" the liver meridian. Kinesiology technique or a Chinese doctor Acupuncturist can help with this.

7. Saying affirmations: I love and support my liver as my liver supports me.
8. Yoga stretches such as: spinal twist (this addresses kidneys and adrenal glands) See your yoga teacher.

Always seek the advice of a professional prior to implementing these suggestions.

YOUR BODY

Detoxing, clearing, increasing awareness, changing habits, moving, swapping, switching, shifting mentally or physically.

CHECK LIST

- Breathing - Deep long slow breaths.
- Affirmations: I am changing, my health is improving every day, my energy is increasing and I am happy.
- Pineal Gland (Sleep regulator) Balance, 10 min morning sun on the forehead. View my Youtube clip.
- Thymus tap: With one hand using rhythm tap your thymus gland on your sternum for a count of 50 especially when you are feeling tired, slow or not well.
- Stress relief balance: Holding forehead with one hand and rubbing K27 located under both sides of your clavicle bone with the other hand while saying your affirmation. Example: My body is relaxed, my liver is working well, I am now very flexible and energetic, and all is well.
- Visualize: Actually visualize yourself exercising, twisting, stretching, moving and even dancing (15 to 30 minutes per day)

- Stretch: Slowly and consciously stretch and move with slow and wave like motions all areas of your body paying much attention to the spine and certain areas where you feel restriction. Always stretch without pain. If you are in pain, stop. Use your affirmations during this time.
- Doctors Visits: Please visit your medical practitioner and discuss, inform and establish an open relationship. Have your blood checked, liver function, thyroid and cholesterol checks etc.
- Visit your Naturopath: Discuss vitamins and supplements such as magnesium, zinc, Fish oil, Co Q150, selenium, Vitamin D, possibly vit C injections.
- Showers: When showering use your cleansing affirmations. (Feng Shui-wise bathrooms represent cleansing and letting go of the old to make way for the new) Re-arrange your bathroom to reflect this affirmation.

WATER

Water is very important. Earth is mostly water and we as humans start with a 90% + percentage of water which makes up our whole body weight. However it reduces as we get older.

So it stands to reason that it would be beneficial for us to pay a lot more attention to the major substance we are made of.

Our bodies are like a battery and the battery fluid being the water is the conductor of where the electrical current passes. These currents carry messages; in our body those messages can be in the form of hormones.

The quality as well as the quantity is very important.

Quantity, time after time I keep getting the message that when we notice we are thirsty it means our body is already dehydrated. So if we form a habit of drinking regularly during the day, this will stabilize this effect. You may like to use a water reminder on your phone until you form the regular habit. Then it will be a natural process. If you are on a raw diet, you will find that your body feels that it is much more hydrated.

CFS sufferers are said to be stuck in a stressed mode. Stress depletes the body of water, so water becomes essential.

When I have a headache, my naturopath advices me to take 2 glasses of water before reaching for pain relief tablets. I would also reach for the hot and cold packs for the liver as well and a good lie down, stay still and relax and let the body heal itself.

Water quality is as important as the quantity, preferably free of chemicals, bacteria, mould, fungus and the right ph balance.

I love Dr Emoto's work, such an inspiration and his devotion to showing us the most essential part of us "water" is simply amazing.

As our body is mostly water, we must be aware of our thoughts and the impact our thought have on our body. As well as what we expose ourselves to, whether it's environmental, chemical, vibrational (such as music), emotional etc.

ALKALINE WATER/DIET

An alkaline ph reading between 6.8 and 7.2 is believed to be the optimal range our body's fluids need to be for it to function at full capacity. Blood PH range (7.35 to 7.45) below or above, this could mean symptoms and disease. If the ph is much below 6.8 or above 7.8 cells it may be malfunctioning. Ideally the reading is 7.4 therefore slightly alkaline.

Ph is the abbreviation for potential hydrogen. The higher the pH reading, the more alkaline and oxygen rich the fluid is. The lower the ph, the more acidic and oxygen deprived the fluids become.

The following is extracted from the following website: www.altered-states.net . The pH in the human digestive tract varies greatly. The pH of saliva is usually between 6.5 - 7.5. After we chew and swallow food it then enters the fundus or upper portion of the stomach which has a pH between 4.0 - 6.5. This is where "pre-digestion" occurs while the lower portion of the stomach is secreting hydrochloric acid (HCI) and pepsin until it reaches a pH between 1.5 - 4.0. The mixture then enters the duodenum (small intestine) where the pH changes to 7.0 - 8.5. This is where 90% of the absorption of nutrients is taken in by the body while the waste products are passed out through the colon (pH 4.0 - 7.0).

If you have a health problem, you are most likely acidic. Research shows that unless the body's pH level is slightly alkaline, the body cannot heal itself. So, no matter what mode you choose to use to take care of your health problem, it won't be completely effective until the pH level is raised. If your body's pH is not balanced, you cannot effectively assimilate vitamins, minerals and food supplements. Your body pH affects everything.

This website explains what is to be believed the process that may not be functioning correctly when CFS and Fibromyalgia occurs view www.altered-states.net.

In my experience with CFS it has been imperative to pay attention to my ph balance, whether it's with foods or with water, ideally both.

CHECK LIST

- Drink water.
- Drink alkaline water.
- Filter your water.
- Use shower/bath water filters.
- Geopathic stress lines/ Ley lines, not sleeping on crossing ley lines.
- Take baths with Epson Salts. (helps with muscle spasms)
- Use bicarb soda regularly.
- Gargle morning and night with Himalayan salt or/and Zeolite Powder.
- MOST important: take colonics regularly.

YOUR ENVIRONMENT

Includes where we live - our environment, home, office, town, surrounding our food, what we see, feel, smell, sense, touch, taste.

There are things we cannot see, or even notice, but as we become more and more sensitive due to this CFS and fibromyalgia and chemical sensitivity, we undeniably become more aware of our environment.

This subject could have an entire book dedicated to it. However, I would like to highlight your awareness with the following check list:

CHECK LIST

- Mould
- Fungus and spores
- Pesticides and Fertilizers
- Ventilation and air quality
- Perfumes
- Chemicals in foods and cleaning products
- EMF's
- Pillows (put out to sun drench regularly) also blankets and your shoes (remember we absorb through our skin, feet and hands).
- Geopathic stress lines, ley lines
- Take regular Epson salt baths (or foot baths)
- Remove plastics from the kitchen area.
- Feng Shui house especially bedroom (remove stressful paintings, objects, colours distracting things from your environment)
- Music, that uplifts and also use to reduce stress.
- Colour Therapy, e.g.: red shoes and red belt (your feet represent your direction and the belt area is where your kidneys and adrenal glands are) may increase energy in these areas.
- Grounding: Very important to release excess negative ions (static) and walk on the grass for at least 5 minutes every day, earth yourself, like any electrical conduit, we do not need excess.
- House clearing: regarding spirits/ ghosts etc.

FOOD

Becoming food focused can be the most essential foundation you can establish.

Improving your health starts with improving the quality and quantity of your food intake.

Food scientists have developed foods that have increased shelf life for our demanding convenience but have not enhanced our health needs.

Optimally we need to eat organic, in season fruit and vegetables.

Shopping regularly for fresh fruit and vegetables could now be the focus on this quest to improve health.

CHECK LIST

- Shop for organic fresh fruit and vegetables
- Preservative free food
- Reduce or omit Genetically Modified foods
- Make sure your fruit and vegetables are in season and decompose quickly, if they last more than a week in your fridge there is something wrong.
- Eating raw 70% of the time. Raw will be your new savior for your gut flora. Greens are the priority.
- Drink fresh green juices. Alkalize quickly.
- Eating fruit and vegetables that have anti-viral and anti-bacterial qualities such as coconuts and pawpaw.
- Yogurt, acidophilus and bifidobacterium preferably coconut yogurt
- Release sugar

- Releasing wheat
- Releasing dairy
- garlic but check sensitivity (allergy testing)
- (REMEMBER THIS DIETRY ADVICE IS EDUCATIONAL ONLY. SEEK THE ADVICE OF YOUR NUTRITIONIST)

IMPROVE YOUR GUT FUNCTION AND YOU COULD IMPROVE YOUR SYMPTOMS OF CFS.

Learn, read, and research what you can do to improve your gut flora. You will also find it will improve your brain function.

Gingko Biloba: is one of those super herbs for CFS clients. It can assist with brain function; however, it needs to be taken with the advice of your naturopath as it is contraindicated if taking blood thinning agents such as blood pressure medication.

I would suggest you read Liz Lipski PhD information on gut function and Leaky gut syndrome. CFS sufferers would greatly benefit from repairing your gut function.

Chapter 9

THE ENERGY KEYS

How I visualise the Chronic Fatigue Syndrome sufferer; Their body looks like a colander, full of holes and less like a solid pot, as it's meant to be.

They are leaking energy.

In this chapter we explore the way we leak energy, emotional as well as physical energy, psychic (the etheric body), the soul and the spirit, whatever you would like to call the energy that we don't usually see. How to notice your sensitivities, energy drains, energy lifters, different types of energy and things that can drain the body of energy. When you are well, being sensitive is not so much an issue but when you are feeling unwell, it is important to take care of yourself and conserve as much energy as possible to allow the body to repair.

The KEY is finding what makes you feel better and what does not.

For example, getting stressed will be easy. Finding what stresses you out is sometimes not so easy. My suggestion here is to get to know yourself on a deeper level.

DEVELOPING YOUR SELF AWARENESS

You have now experienced chronic fatigue syndrome's symptoms and felt the changes into becoming a sensitive person. You may have noticed sensitivity not only emotionally but physically. You may experience many sensitivities, such as: Sensitivity to light, sound, tastes, smells, touch, music, vibrations, radiation, radio waves, ley lines, chemicals, additives, wheat, dairy, coffee, alcohol, perfumes and colours in the environment.

When looking at the physical aspect in the loss of energy, we can refer to something such as infections for example. Where emotional drains are referring to the affect that you may have as a result of dealing with negative people, for example. After being with these people for awhile, you may feel a definite inclination to go and rest or you may feel heavy or simply drained of energy. This can happen to healthy people too, but to the Chronic Fatigue sufferer it is very important to limit the time spent with people who demand your attention and energy. You will be able to identify these people quite easily, no matter how much time you spend with them, you are never left with a feeling of being uplifted and light or happy. Sometimes these people dump a great deal of responsibility on you without you noticing. They may ask you to do things that you are clearly in no position to commit to. They usually do not see how you feel they are too involved in getting what they want out of you, and anyone else for that matter. They are used to you being well and doing what you want them to do.

INFECTIONS

When the gut lining is inflamed it is believed that the body is unable to ward off bacteria, viruses and parasites as well as fungus and yeast like Candida, with ease. These pathogens then pass from the gut cavity to the bloodstream and set up infection anywhere else in the body.

This could be an important theory, regarding loss of energy for the CFS sufferer, because the body is constantly having to deal with underlying infections somewhere in the body. This could take up a great deal of energy to produce the white blood cells necessary to clean up infections.

ENERGY DRAINS

For you to be able to return to a strong, healthy lifestyle, it is necessary for you to be aware of your energy drains, starting with likes and dislikes. This is a specialized skill that you will master and come to rely on to avoid your energy draining.

EXERCISE: AWARENESS SKILL

Sit in front of a picture which you may have hanging at home. Ask yourself, what do I like about this picture? It could be the colour, it could be the subject it could be the frame. Ask yourself, how does this picture make me feel? You may like it or you may notice you really do not like it at all but have not noticed it before. If you don't like the picture, remove it. Start changing things that do not make you feel good. Sometimes we are surrounded by things that drain us but we simply ignore them.

That was your first step to re-prioritizing your whole life.

Now let's look at other things in your life, from what you wear, what you wash with, what you eat, what you expose yourself to everyday, or even to whom you expose yourself to.

It's not an easy process and it can be a real eye opener. I feel that because of the huge energy drain on the body that comes with this syndrome, the ability to focus on some of your basic needs and wants tends to fall by the wayside. This alone can have a cumulative effect. You start to put up with things that simply are not beneficial for you because you don't have the energy to think about it, or do something, about changing it.

Making a list of all your stressors is essential.

STRESS LIST

When looking at things that can be described as stress, note that stress on the body can come from different areas and situations. It may be helpful to view it as, what makes your body weak.

Here are some examples of situations where stress could manifest from. You could section them into these 4 categories:

Categories:

1. SELF
2. OTHERS
3. CIRCUMSTANCES
4. THINGS

EXAMPLES: Situations

Allergies
Anxiety
Boss
Not enough money/work load
Negative self talk
Brother/sister
Just being ill
Addicted to some foods/drink/etc
Office bully
Chemicals/cleaning products

ENERGY LIFTERS

Next we are looking into what makes you happy and strong. Think carefully about all the things that make you feel good. Making a list of energy lifters may be more important than the Stress List.

Categories:

1. SELF
2. OTHERS
3. CIRCUMSTANCES
4. THINGS

EXAMPLES:

Painting
Going out with friends
Traveling

Reading/watching movies
Dancing
Walking dog
Helping people
family
getting a massage
music

BOUNDARIES

Set your emotional and personal boundaries.

Example: One of my personal boundaries: Do not talk to a particular family member for more than I have to because she upsets me. My energy gets disrupted and I feel weak.

Set your boundaries, make them clear. Excuse yourself and leave. This is not a matter of (I should) it's a matter of I NEED TO DO THIS! If you don't, you will possibly become ill and spend some days in bed.

Once you understand and accept what your boundaries are, taking action by changing things to accommodate your new boundaries will be easier. Here are some examples of boundaries:

SAY NO OFTEN.

Can you say no effectively?

Can you say no loudly? If you can't do this comfortably, then this is definitely something you need to practice. Here is an idea, why not practice it in the car? When you are driving, while no one can hear you yelling, say out loud,"No! No I do not want to, no I do not like that, no I do not care for that, no it's not my style, no I am not happy with that, no it does not really interest me, no, thank you, may be next time.

Also use different tones of voice and pitches, see how you feel when you change the sound of the same sentence.

Do you say no, but then notice a change in your body when you are trying to please people. Train yourself to say no, and that is final.

If you truly find it difficult, why not try this to start with?

Avoid the answer. You could say: maybe, later, could be, sure, not sure, etc. This can be useful while you are training yourself to say no.

I know the brain does not function as well as it used to and sometimes it's hard to make decisions or even speak up when your energy levels are so low. But I really encourage you to train yourself to say NO!.

Inna Segal author of 'The secret language of your body' talks about Chronic Fatigue and feeling stuck, resisting life, not knowing how to say no, ignoring your body and much more. If you get a chance, do not pass up reading her book, it was fascinating and I cannot recommend it highly enough.

I know I have to work on this, I am better now but it's still an issue I am working on.

EMOTIONAL ASPECT OF INFLAMMATION

Looking at the emotional side or connection to inflammation, Annette Noontil and Inna Segal, have the following insights on inflammation from a spiritual aspect or emotional take:

Irritation, inner conflict, aggravation. Seething inside and feeling undermined. Irrational, angry at the injustice you are seeing or experiencing. Allowing others to control and dominate you. Self-sabotage.

I certainly can relate to many of these aspects, and it will be very interesting to see how many of them you may also relate.

How I view these emotions: They are a sign for you to take responsibility for feeling this way. It is not always about how you feel, but it can also be that you may be watching someone dear to you experiencing these aspects of emotions and it can manifest an effect on your own body or thoughts.

It also could be about circumstances or things. For example looking at injustice, it could be about the injustice you saw somewhere and collected strong emotions towards something that happened to someone else or to a building or an animal for example.

EMOTIONAL ASPECT OF INFECTION

These emotions include feeling attacked, invaded, chaotic, irritated, annoyed, threatened, and weakened. Letting down your defenses, feeling vulnerable needing attention and rest.

How this information is used is up to you. I will, however, make note that emotions are extremely powerful information that our bodies show us. As you learn to read accept and work on the release of them, they become powerful tools that help us to grow as well as heal.

Emotions have been the best tools I have noticed and experienced so far, in the human being, to guide us through healing. They are like short burst of electrical current that alerts us.

When an emotion comes up and we notice it because it either takes us by surprise or you simply acknowledge the emotion, it is the bodies red flags to stop and listen. Just like pain is to the physical body.

TAKING ACTION WITH FUN

Having fun is essential, scientifically speaking, for a person with Chronic Fatigue Syndrome so planning for "Fun things to do" even if it's a short activity. It's better to use your adrenaline in this powerful way which will decrease your cortisol levels than doing the "I have to or I should" activities.

If you can master the energy to do an activity that you truly find fun, even though you know it will take energy, do it anyway. It will change your neurological pattern as well as release good hormones, which in turn, the body will replenish these hormones, as a chain reaction. Some people get addicted to bike riding, weight lifting, running, swimming, etc because they get hooked on the adrenaline hormone the body produces by these activities, described as the feel good hormone.

We need to somehow build up this feel good hormone again because it is very low in Chronic fatigue sufferers. Cortisol in the morning, for example there seems to be a correlation between low levels and chronic fatigue.

CORTISOL

Some relevant information on CORTISOL and why it's important for CFS sufferers.

Cortisol is an important hormone in the body secreted by the adrenal glands and is involved in the following functions and more:

- proper glucose metabolism
- regulation of blood pressure
- insulin release for blood sugar maintenance
- immune function
- inflammatory response

Generally, its levels are higher in the body in the morning and decrease at night. Even though stress is not the only thing that makes the body secrete cortisol, it has been connected and referred to as "the stress hormone" because it is secreted during the "fight flight" response to stress. It is also responsible for several stress related changes in the body. Small increases of cortisol have some positive effects like:

a quick burst of energy for survival reasons
heightened memory functions
a burst of increased immunity
lower sensitivity to pain
helps maintain homeostasis in the body

In thinking about cortisol I wonder if it keeps getting released and we don't have the proper mechanism intact to stop the cortisol from releasing itself. Could it be that we are not repairing and regaining the cortisol levels necessary to function properly?

Cortisol is important and helps the body to cope with stress, but the body also needs to return to normal and the relaxation response needs to kick in. Except it seems that in our high stress culture, or maybe due to other things that we have not, as yet, been aware of, the body does not always have a chance to return to normal, resulting in a state of chronic stress.

In the theories section I write about my belief that sometimes a state of chronic stress is created possibly as a reaction, allergy to or even damage caused to the adrenal gland by the use of synthetic adrenaline (Epinephrine). These are administered in drugs such as anesthetics. The body's stress response is activated so often, that it does not have a chance to return to normal and therefore creates chronic stress.

Cortisol and adrenaline (epinephrine) hormones come from the adrenal glands, interestingly they are not only hormones but neurotransmitters because they function by carrying the nerve impulses between the neurons to the cells.

Cortisol helps the liver to detox, it heightens short term memory and an anti-inflammatory.

Our bodies need to have these two hormones balanced.

Factors that generally decrease cortisol levels.

- magnesium supplements
- Omega 3
- Music therapy
- Massage therapy
- Laughing therapy
- Crying (after a stressful situation)

- Dancing
- Vitamin C
- Black tea

Factors that generally increase cortisol levels.

- Caffeine
- Sleep deprivation
- Prolonged physical exercise
- Hypo-estrogenism and melatonin supplementation increase cortisol levels in post-menopausal women.
- Burn out, or severe trauma or stressful event or grief
- Anorexia nervosa
- Contraceptive Pill
- Commuting (long distances in the car)
- I am sure medication, poisoning, allergies, and anything else that lowers or interferes with the immune response could play a part in this.

(The following is extracted from: http://www.endo-society.org.) Dr. Wilson, the "stress" doctor and world authority on fatigue, stress and adrenal function actually coined the phrase "adrenal fatigue" in 1998. Dr. Wilson found through his extensive research spanning over 30 years that there is almost no part of the body which is not affected to some degree by cortisol.

The following study highlights the importance of salivary cortisol testing correlating with fatigue and appeared in the March 2008 issue of JCEM, Journal of Clinical Endocrinology & Metabolism, one of the four journals published by The Endocrine Society.

People who suffer from chronic fatigue syndrome (CFS) often endure months of persistent fatigue, muscle pain, and impaired memory and concentration. Understanding the physiological changes that accompany CFS, however, has been difficult, but a new study accepted for publication in the Journal of Clinical Endocrinology & Metabolism (JCEM) reveals that abnormally low morning concentrations of the hormone cortisol produced by the adrenal glands, may be correlated with more severe fatigue in CFS patients, especially in women.

"We're learning more and more about the complexities of the illness that is chronic fatigue syndrome," said William C. Reeves, M.D., with the Centers for Disease Control and Prevention in Atlanta, Georgia, and lead author of the study. "This research helps us draw a clearer picture in regards to how CFS affects people, which ultimately will lead to more effective management of patients with CFS."

For their study, the researchers screened 19,381 residents of Georgia, selecting 292 people who had CFS, 268 who were considered chronically unwell, and 163 who were considered well to participate. The researchers then measured free cortisol concentrations in saliva, which was collected on regular workdays, immediately upon awaking and 30 minutes and 60 minutes after awakening. The data indicated different profiles of cortisol concentrations over time among the groups, with the CFS group showing an attenuated morning cortisol profile.

Study participants were purposely screened and enrolled from the community, rather than from volunteers identified at a specialty referral clinic. The purpose of this study design was to provide results that would be more generalized to the population suffering from CFS.

In this study, women with CFS exhibited significantly lower morning cortisol profiles when compared with well women.

This study confirms previous research indicating that CFS is related to an imbalance in the normal interactions among the various systems of the body that work together to manage stress. "People with CFS have reduced overall cortisol output within the first hour after they wake up in the morning, which is actually one of the most stressful times for the body," Dr. Reeves said. "We need further studies to better understand the relationship between morning cortisol levels and functional status of a patient suffering from CFS."

Founded in 1916, The Endocrine Society is the world's oldest, largest, and most active organization devoted to research on hormones, and the clinical practice of endocrinology. Today, The Endocrine Society's membership consists of over 14,000 scientists, physicians, educators, nurses and students in more than 80 countries. Together, these members represent all basic, applied, and clinical interests in endocrinology. To learn more about the Society, and the field of endocrinology, visit www.endo-society.org.

I found this research fascinating and noteworthy and would encourage you to pursue the understanding of this hormone in reference to your own symptoms of CFS. It may be a good idea to speak to your doctor and naturopath about checking your cortisol and adrenaline levels. I would suggest you download Dr Myhill's book where she details what type of medical tests you can ask for.

I have observed in relation to cortisol signs and symptoms in the body, that when I started to get better, especially when I ate a raw food diet, my inflammation in the gut changed and a whole list of symptoms started to disappear. These included, sore muscles, hot and restless legs, nausea, headaches, memory improved, my sleep was deeper, I woke up feeling strong, my sugar cravings were gone and I did not have that dip in energy when I did something that used a lot of energy. I also had changes to my skin and lymph.

Wise words from Rosanna Commisso.

"Chi is energy. Energy is necessary for life. What are the benefits of having healthy free flowing Chi?

It's what gives you your spark and keeps you firing on all cylinders. To be healthy, your Chi must be plentiful and circulate easily. If your Chi is weak or becomes blocked, problems will arise. So it makes sense to strengthen your Chi and work on improving its circulation through diet, Chi exercises, your environment as well as your thoughts.

All living things carry Chi energy. This includes the food you eat. The following Chi food principles can guide you towards a diet that restores your body's natural, self-healing abilities by increasing your Chi.

Organically Grown: Eat fresh organic locally grown produce, as these are very high in natural Chi.

In Season: Eat according to the season. In winter eat more pressure-cooked grains, roots and hearty soups, while in summer cook less and eat more salads. The Chi in food is affected by the seasons, so you want your food to support the Chi around you.

Natural: Avoid refined processed high-stress foods containing preservatives, artificial colors and flavors that delete Chi.

Locally Grown: If grown locally and in season the nature of the food's Chi should be in tune with the Chi of the local environment and is more likely to meet the body's needs.

Raised in the Wild: When possible choose meats, poultry and fish that has been raised in the wild as this means that their Chi will be high.

Mood: In order to utilize the Chi in your food, make sure you are relaxed when eating. Irregular eating, skipping meals and eating on the run or while upset will deplete your Stomach and Spleen Chi.

80% Rule: For optimal Chi, eat until you are 80% full. Too much food can disorder Chi, not enough food weakens your Chi. Eating too much causes stagnation in the meridians. Food stagnation leads to internal heat and damp phlegm which together can cause bloating, restlessness, gas, fatigue, a heavy sensation in the body, skin infections or canker sores.

Balance of Flavors: Ensure that your meals contain a combination of the five flavors; sweet, sour, bitter, spicy and salty. Each flavour has a certain effect on your body, so it's important to ensure that they are balanced. The energy from sour-tasting food (vinegar, yoghurt and many herbs) have an affinity with the liver meridian, bitter foods to the heart, sweet to the spleen, pungent flavours like ginger and spices relate to the lung and salt to the kidney meridian.

Hydration: Water is vital for life and for the creation of Chi, so make sure you replenish this daily.

Time: The best time to eat a large meal is between 7am-11am, as this is when your Stomach and Spleen Chi is at its most powerful.

Cooking Methods: The way in which food is cooked also affects its Chi. Your particular imbalance will determine the best cooking method for you. However, microwaving is not recommended as it creates internal dryness and weakens your Stomach and Spleen Chi.

Balance Yin & Yang: All life on earth balances two complementary and opposite natural forces: expansion and contraction or yin and yang. Contraction holds our bodies together while expansive forces enable us to breathe, move around, think and feel. To stay in good health your body needs to keep both forces in balance. To do this you need to eat a balance of both expansive and contractive foods.

If you feel heavy, slow, hot, tense, sluggish, constipated, frustrated, irritable or too intense, you need to eat more Yin or expansive food such as fruit, honey, milk, yogurt and salads.

If you have sweet cravings, energy bursts followed by fatigue, cold hands and feet, no will power, feel moody, dreamy, spaced out or confused, irregular bowels, recurring colds and infections, you need to eat more Yang or contractive foods such as cheese, eggs, meat, nuts and tuna.

With an understanding of Chi, Yin/Yang and the meridians, you will be able to choose foods that are appropriate for your particular need.

By following these simple, yet powerful tips, you can increase your energy and improve your health by facilitating your Chi.

(ArticlesBase SC #1762818)

About the Author:

Rosanna Commisso has been practicing yoga for over 25 years. She studied both Hatha and Ki Yoga. In addition to her love of yoga, Rosanna brings with her over 20 years experience working in both the traditional and alternative health sectors as a hospital pharmacist, counsellor and natural health educator. Rosanna developed ChiYo after being diagnosed with CFS and adrenal fatigue and wanting to find a form of exercise that would help heal, revive, energize and calm her body. Her goal was to create a class that would benefit anyone looking for a restorative practice.

As you can appreciate, the research that goes into finding the best available information or information that can stimulate and form faith in healing from chronic fatigue syndrome is out there. The problem we all face with chronic fatigue syndrome's symptoms is a lack of energy to keep digging and finding these treasures and the energy to employ what resonates with us. I hope these chapters are stimulating your own drive to research into ways you can heal.

Chapter 10

BUDGETING FOR CHRONIC ILLNESS

One of the main priorities is to come to terms with the demands of your chronic symptoms. You will need to establish the areas of your life that this health situation is affecting now and could impact in the future. How much money you will be investing on which part of the illness that you find is most important to achieve a release of symptom which could have a financial improvement on your life.

How to break down the priorities:

SYMPTOMS

Chronic
Brain fog
Pain
Neck Pain

Mild
Sleep deprived
Nausea
Headaches

Comes and goes
Really bad days collapse days
Tinnitus
Body strength

Looking at the above examples, we would first identify what our symptoms are and where on the grid we are at the moment. Then we can identify what our current personal goal is. Your personal goal could be just to get to work and back in one piece. Or it could be releasing the frustration of brain fog. That might be the issue that could be stopping you from doing many activities, simply because it is hard to focus. Remember short and long term memory dysfunction effects are connected to brain fog. Sometimes brain fog can be just that feeling of being in a cloud.

Example No.1: brain fog

Brain fog can make it very difficult to concentrate, to make decisions, to research your illness, to communicate with people and to simply get your needs met.

Ask yourself how does this affect me on a scale of one to ten? With No. 1 indicating low and would point out this does not affect me at all, through to the highest score, No. 10 – indicating this is currently having a significant effect on me and my life.

This may also vary from day to day, even hour to hour.

My suggestion to reduce brain fog:

Delete wheat, dairy and sugar from your diet.

Do colonics fortnightly or weekly (depending on what you can manage)

Repair gut function. (see chapter on gut function)

Budgeting for chronic illness is not easy, and everyone's budgets are different. My personal suggestion is not necessarily for everyone and what I put at the top of my priority list may not be your most urgent item to tackle. But, if I chose brain fog as being my priority, you could go to the doctors and ask for all the tests possible to establish how my gut is functioning. Read Dr Sarah Myhill's free book on her website drmyhill.co.uk for tests that can be requested from your GP/doctor.

Possibly delete wheat bread and change to spelt bread or even better, go on a raw diet and use cos lettuce instead of bread altogether.

Remove dairy (including butter) for the first 3 months. You can always re-introduce it later.

You could remove sugar from the diet. This is super critical when it comes to reducing brain fog and your gut function. This can also repair any candida issues as well as helping with parasite issues and malabsorbtion of nutrients through the gut wall. It can also help with bowel health.

You could search for the nearest colonic irrigation therapist and speak to them about a possible long term plan and ask for a discount for a 12 month program of their colonic treatments. For example if you decide to do fortnightly for 12 months ask for a sensible discount.

Once your memory starts improving it will make such a difference to your daily life. My suggestion to improve memory is taking the 'Gingko' herbal mix "Liquid" not tablets or capsules. Please take note that gingko is not recommended when taking blood thinning medication such as 'warfarin' or any other blood thinning medical drug. (Warfarin is also known by the brand names Coumadin, Jantoven, Marevan, Uniwarfin, Warf) it is an anticoagulant normally used in the prevention of thrombosis and thromboembolism, the formation of blood clots in the blood vessels and their migration elsewhere in the body respectively.

I classified tinnitus under the mild category so I would not be investing in this unless I had achieved my most important goal which would be brain fog for my choice. Pain and headaches were my next in line to invest in. So I set my financial budget to attend Osteopathic or Physiotherapy appointments and pain relief techniques.

You may find that when your brain function and gut function starts to improve, the tinnitus also improves.

Ways to reduce tinnitus include:

Check your magnesium levels. This can be done via blood tests or hair analysis, which is my preference. A naturopath can take a small sample of your hair and send it off for analysis. This will show the levels of many minerals in your systems. You can also compare these every couple of months and see how your system is improving.

However, you do not always need to test for things to determine if your body needs that particular mineral or supplement. One option is to muscle test for a specific mineral. You can consult a Kinesiologist to test several minerals, products, or even techniques. You can also ask for priorities to find what the body needs at that particular time.

Check your zinc levels, your vitamin B's and C's. When my B levels were low, my doctor arranged blood tests as I had annoying tinnitus at the time. However, since my very strict raw diet the tinnitus reduced and my blood tests now show higher Vitamin B levels. However, once you start eating processed food again the tinnitus may return.

Gingko is an excellent herbal product that I personally use and it is also great for improving memory.

TINNITUS

Speak to your Naturopath about any allergies that you may have, there may be a connection with allergies and tinnitus.

Anti-inflammatory herbs such as Stinging Nettle are also a helpful herb for tinnitus and worth discussing with your naturopath.

With Traditional Chinese Medicine, tinnitus is connected in two meridians, excess liver and kidney deficiency. An acupuncturist can advise you on your situation.

Please note when you are dehydrated your tinnitus can become more prominent.

FRUSTRATIONS AND UNCERTAINTIES

Much has been written about coping with chronic fatigue syndrome. These include keeping a pain diary, tracking your moods, setting goals. Dr Peter Dingle suggestions include:

DIARY

Keep a Pain diary, with dates and description of the type of pain and where in the body it is.

NOTE: this diary is to be used not abused. It is a common problem with CFS patients to panic and form irrational thoughts regarding their pain and symptoms, so if you find you are dwelling on your symptoms put the diary away and only write in it once a month. This is vitally important. It is not meant to stress you out, it is meant to monitor your progress.

In this diary it is also helpful to note allergies that you are discovering whether it is food or things like chemical, preservatives, food colorings, medicine (drugs) etc, that are affecting you. It is very important also to note other types of stress like mental, emotional or over activity. You might include the date and specific incidents that have triggered these emotions.

If you work in an environment like child care, or nursing, massage or other health professions where you are in physical contact with people, this may sometimes become challenging when there are outbreaks of viral and bacterial infections. The end result - to us it means days in bed. Sometimes the usual symptoms of the bug that is going around does not manifest the same way in Chronic Fatigue Syndrome people but what you get is the typical CFS symptoms. These may include aching body, heavy eye lids, glassy eyes, and overwhelming fatigue. This can sometimes feel like you are wearing a lead dental x-ray apron, not to mention the headaches etc. While everyone else might get a sniffle or mucus discharge, we get major CFS symptoms.

MOODS

The mood swings are another classic for CFS sufferers, especially when you're feeling low in energy, weak, headachy, dizzy or confused. I call this the liver scream.

It has a resemblance to hangover moodiness, except without the alcohol. Some people call it liver congestion. The end results - you are left feeling toxic. I understand that some people get very moody, angry and agitated, yelling, screaming, and throwing things. If you do recognize these symptoms, the best thing to do is to put yourself to bed. And you could follow the instructions on the DVD FIRST AID FOR CFS which I have developed to help people during an episode of acute symptoms of CFS.

THE CFS FIRST AID DVD

The DVD has important information on techniques which can help you with an acute episode of CFS. Visit www.chronicfatigueshop.com.au

SETTING HEALTH GOALS

The following information was inspired by the teachings of Dr Peter Dingle.

Make specific goals to change behaviour, whether it's conscious or unconscious.

I always feel it is important to start small. Taking baby steps in a process that you will be using for the rest of your life, because you are building your foundation and behavioural pattern for healthy behavioural change.

STEP ONE

Find the most stressful aspect of your illness.

STEP TWO

Get to know your stress issue by looking at it from different angles; maybe discuss it with your family, friends or doctor. Understand the issue well. Write about it in your journal and use descriptive language to connect with the issue on different levels. If this sounds easy, its not, especially when your cognitive abilities are impaired.

STEP THREE

Form a goal using positive language. For example if my goal is to release brain fog, the language I would use could be something like, I feel clear and decisive, I now enjoy using my memory and feel proud to have achieved this.

STEP FOUR

Reinforce the goal with one or more affirmations (also please note to use positive language)

STEP FIVE

Place your affirmation where you can see it on a regular basis, read it often.

You can also attach a picture to it to reinforce the meaning.

CLIENT PRACTITIONER DISCUSSION LIST

PERSONAL GOALS

What do you really want, think about your values and form what you want taking these into consideration.

When do you want it? Be precise and set a specific time frame to achieve your goals.

How will you get it? Make up at least 10 smaller specific steps; these are the strategies and tasks.

Why do you want it? Get personal here, really get into your values and keep adding to this list.

Who will help you get there? Who can support, motivate you, give you feedback.

Where will you do it from? Find a place to inspire you, a supportive positive environment. Could be CFS support groups.

Where is it taking you? Think where you are going with this, always fit your goals into a long term vision.

NOTE: You need to budget to either spend time with a caretaker or family member, or a practitioner to help you with some of these activities. I do understand with CFS you are likely to struggle with cognitive exercises. And that is where you need to work out where you will be investing your money on.

The following is Dr Peter Dingle's article on goals.

Beyond Goals Dr Peter Dingle and Terry Power –

Author of Goal Getting. The Science of setting successful goals.

Over the last 20 years I've given many people information on how to improve their health and the environment, running seminars and even one on one sessions, and I've come to the realisation that there are big gaps between what people want to do and what they actually do. So just over 10 years ago I started researching goal setting for healthy behavioural change. I realised that even after the best possible seminar and motivational session it was only the goal setters who actually carried through with the necessary changes. Without goals most of the information was wasted and in some cases extra information was even detrimental, as it made people feel quite overwhelmed. I now build in goal setting with all the groups I take, including high school kids, teachers, community groups and sporting and business teams. With my research students I've worked on programs such as Travel Smart, developed the program Living Smart and the latest, on which we're currently working, is Seniors Smart. And of course I use goal setting extensively in my own personal life.

Having goals is fundamental to human behaviour. It's not just for sports people and business people; it's for anyone who wants to improve their life. In fact goal setting begins in early childhood and stays with us for the rest of our lives. Setting and achieving goals is not just an important process, it is essential to our lives. It plays a major role in personality, motivation and health. Hence my focus on goal setting as a fundamental aspect of wellbeing. Our studies have shown that when you begin to succeed in achieving your goals (and they may be any goals, not specifically related to health) your health will begin to improve as there is a transference effect.

The research on the positive effects of goal setting is overwhelming. In a recent review, researchers who had been studying the effect of setting goals for the past 35 years found that goal setting increased performance on well over 100 tasks involving more than 40,000 participants, in at least 8 different countries, working in laboratory, simulation and field settings, in time spans from one minute to 25 years. They reported that the results are applicable not only to individuals, but to groups, organisational units and organisations. In effect the review found that goal setting is amongst the most valid and practical applications for motivation in psychology.

My own review of more than 600 peer review journals on goals and the writing of my book 'Goal Getting' with Terry Power, shows without doubt that having goals does work. They are an incredibly effective tool, whether you wish to improve your health and well being or family life, or your finances or sporting ability. The research shows that if you set your goals well, then you'll be successful in achieving them. Behaviour modification programs which incorporate goal setting are significantly more effective and have more consistent results than any other type of intervention. In a program designed to increase dietary fibre consumption, those who set goals consumed 91 per cent more fibre than the people who didn't set goals. Goal setting is probably the single most important factor in a successful diet or weight loss program. Will power is what you rely on if you have a wish that you have not made into a goal, and often only works till 3 pm the next day when you are tired, hungry and confront your first major challenge. Goals take you beyond the limits of your will power.

Goals don't work for people mainly because they simply don't set them well. In some cases they have literally never thought about it, so their goals are just a loose bunch of dreams or wishes, much like a wish list for Father Christmas. But even those people who have read a book or attended a course on goal setting don't necessarily succeed because they have not been taught to set goals comprehensively and thoroughly enough. The most common reason people don't succeed, is that they don't write their goals down and they don't work on them. Finally, goals don't work in isolation from the rest of the universe and everything else you do, so you need to think beyond your goals and build in an additional battery of support. If your goals are worthwhile, and they should be, what other forms of cognitive behaviour therapy can you use to support your goals? For example, I have people tell me that their goals never work for them or that they have no imagination. Yes, I get people who really believe this. So they need additional techniques such as establishing a positive mental dialogue or Emotional Freedom Techniques to get them over their first barrier. Otherwise they won't even be in the race.

Goals work because they focus our thoughts, gives us the tools to do the job and motivate us to keep going. Goals are not just a single thought about what you want - they are a comprehensive and ongoing process. To set meaningful goals, which you'll want to achieve.

I have seen many goal programs that don't cover these questions in any depth, remember the old adage: "The bluntest pencil records better than the sharpest mind."

A last word on goals: make them fun and pertinent. Start by developing your goals in areas that excite you and/or are fun. If you like reading, develop your goals around reading, and you will find it will help you set goals in many other areas of your life! Or if you have a penchant for a particular sport or hobby, set your goals so that you integrate that interest area. One young boy I was working with wanted to be a jockey, so the first goal we set was that he was an excellent jockey and he was getting better. Out of that came the fact that it's a physically demanding job, so we needed to set some health goals. He needed a good diet so he'd have the necessary energy and stamina, and so on. Goals should be interesting!" End of quote look up the website Dr Dingle . com for the full article.

I hope this emphasis on goals comes across because it makes a huge difference in tackling the many tasks that a person with CFS has to put together to achieve results in releasing their symptoms.

Chapter 11

PAIN

Pain relief is important when pain becomes prominent in your life. The usual pharmacological, temporary products available are just that, not for long term consumption.

Taking care of your pain long term takes strength of character and determination and of course faith that this pain will stop one day. Many people become fixated and use much of their energy thinking that the pain will never go away, especially when this pain is present for more than 2 years. However the more you talk about the pain, the more you actively engage your whole day around the pain, by making appointments with physicians, physiotherapist, and other professionals, the more emphasis you are giving the pain.

Making plans to manage the pain is important, just as important as making an affirmation of what your life will look like when you no longer have pain. Giving this visualisation and affirmation as much time and effort as you give the appointments to physicians will break the negative pattern. An affirmation I use often is: thank you for my healing, my body feels strong and healthy. The energy weight that this affirmation carries may assist in balancing the pain.

MUSCLE PAIN RELIEF

Karyl's tips

- Yoga stretches: Become familiar with Yoga and maybe to some classes, not only does Yoga work on the differ muscle groups but also works on the meridian pathwa I believe that the central spinal fluid becomes gel like a when your body moves it can creak and crackle and becor very congested. The more you move the better the spine flu becomes. You may notice the crackle noises become less ar the range of movement is much much better with stretchin
- Epson salts (Magnesium) body baths and foot baths regularl For muscle pain.
- My naturopath recommends: Ultra Muscle Eze, which is a magnesium and multi vitamin complex (Magnesium relaxes muscles) this particular brand is by Metagenics, but there are others on the market.
- Remedial Massage for the relief of muscle spasms and cramps. (Note: I would not recommend a full 1 hour massage when you are not well it makes the symptoms worse. As I believe that it may push the toxins through the body, even though in 2 to 3 days you feel better some sensitive people get concerned)
- Herbal mix : Relaxing herbs like valerium, passionfruit flower.
- Homeopathics like Hypericum, nux vormica, chamomile, rhus tox, arnica, I am a big user of these homeopathics and I find benefit from them, there are other homeopathics, in which your homeopath or naturopath can help you with.
- Vitamin B, even Berrocca is great.

- There are magnesium injections and vitamin B injections that your doctor can give you. (I found these did not have an impact on my every day pain levels but I am not ruling out that it could help some of you).
- Resting is also a great simple thing to do. Staying very very still and take deep breaths allows the oxygen to be carried throughout the body and it allows the body to use energy for healing organs and body structures, instead of using the energy for muscle contractions in walking for example. Meditate and reduce your anxiety levels so you can allow the body to heal the affected area.
- I recommend the affirmation: Thank you for my healing, I alway say this as a mantra especially when I am sick, it instantly calms me down and allows the healing to work.
- Breath into the pain. As you breath out visualize breathing out the pain and the germs.
- Colour therapy, imagine the healing colour of yellow on the particular area that is causing you pain thank the body for the pain signals and accept and release the pain, using your breath. Stay still and do not ignore these signals they are there for a reason.
- Earthing yourself is a must, I feel. We are energy beings who carry magnetic and electrical current. Go outside and put your feet on the ground for at least 20 minutes. On the grass, dirt, rock what ever is available. It can discharge your body from excess electricity and earth your body. If you can not go outside for what ever reason I would think about getting an earthing mat, this uses the earthing current of your house to earth you. Search the net or youtube for these products.

- Temporary relief sometimes can be found with Panadol, and other paracetamol products, however not always, especially if you have nausea with it and it feels more like a liver connected pain. (The hangover nausea, pain) Many times Panadol did not help me at all. Hot and cold packs on the liver did. So thats 2 minutes cold pack on the liver and 10 minutes hotpack and alternate for about 20 minutes at a time, do it 2 or 3 times per day.

VAGUS NERVE RESPONSE

While in a good deal of pain, having 2 neck cervical slipped discs and nerve impingement, I sought the help of an Osteopath and later a physiotherapist. My experience with the Vagus Nerve Response was horrible and frightening, everyone else was quite blazzae about it.

I was getting a treatment from the Osteopath on my neck, and I felt he was quite rough and quick with his corrections this particular time. I was feeling very vulnerable, sensitive at the time and with the usual fibromyalgic body pain. When I sat up on the treatment table the room went dark, I could not see the Osteopath's face everything started spinning, I felt nausea and a massive thumping headache, I wanted to vomit, I felt so sick. I said to him where is the bucket I can't see anything and I need to vomit. The Osteopath said don't worry its just a Vagus Nerve Response.

It frightened me and his lack of empathy was so annoying, a drink of water would have been the minimum I myself as a practitioner, would have done in that circumstance, all he said is relax and sit outside before you drive home. Well, I could hardly see in front of me. I was not wanting to kill anyone with my car, so I sat in the car for over 1/2 hour and drank my bottle of water. It did settle down and eventually I drove home and rested for the remainder of the day.

Not to this extent but a similar reaction I experienced also with a treatment from the physiotherapist, except he was much kinder and gave me a glass of water and spoke to me about this reaction. My questions to him was; can you take my blood pressure?, maybe my bp went down too quickly with the pain reaction. He did not have one available. I have a high pain threshold as well as being very sensitive to products etc. I had noticed that since I have reduced my stress from a particular relationship source my central nervous system has responded very well and my recovery has improved significantly from stress stimuli. I had another reaction similar but not to the same extent when I was having blood tests, they needed 9 viles and when he got to 7, I started getting dizzy and unwell, wanted to vomit, similar to the suspected Vagus Nerve Reactions. Oh the joys of the weird and wonderful world of the CFS sufferers. The doctors comments, no idea, yep could be a Vagus Nerve Reaction. Make sure you are well hydrated before you go for treatments or blood tests.

Gee, this business of not drinking water seems very consequential, I might get a vagus nerve response? Better carry your water bottles if you have had this lovely experience with Vagus Nerve responses.

Some info on Vagus Nerve response: wiki: Activation of the vagus nerve typically leads to a reduction in heart rate, blood pressure, or both. This occurs commonly in the setting of gastrointestinal illness such as viral gastroenteritis or acute cholecystitis, or in response to other stimuli, including carotid sinus massage, Valsalva maneuver, or pain from any cause, in particular, having blood drawn. When the circulatory changes are great enough, vasovagal syncope results. Relative dehydration tends to amplify these responses.

Excessive activation of the vagal nerve during emotional stress, which is a parasympathetic overcompensation of a strong sympathetic nervous system response associated with stress, can also cause vasovagal syncope because of a sudden drop in blood pressure and heart rate. Vasovagal syncope affects young children and women more than other groups. It can also lead to temporary loss of bladder control under moments of extreme fear.

Interestingly, since I have healed my gastrointestinal area with a raw food diet and the stressful relationship slowly took left stage, my body has been responding incredibly well, no fibromyalgia pain, increased in strength, great response to painful neck adjustments and a whole list more.

THE AMYGDALA RETRAINING

Dr Ashok Gupta in the Uk has developed this training to relieve symptoms of CFS and Fibromyalgia with his technique, which he calls Gupta Amygdala Retraining Programme. I purchased his DVD and attended his Webinars and found the system to have a significant affect on the reduction of symptoms of CFS and fibromyalgia.

Ashok explains that this treatment is not, cognitive behavioural therapy, reverse therapy, psychotherapy, lightning process, pacing therapy, michel therapy, positive thinking, basic relaxation, hypnosis or hypnotherapy.

It is a drug free therapy, Ashok clearly states that ME/CFS is a real physical condition, with real physical symptoms. This is based on his medical paper which was published in a medical journal in 2002. The explanation is based on the role of a brain structure called the Amygdala, which he believes keeps the body in a permanent imbalanced state, causing all the symptoms.

My sick days were many, better still I will start explaining it backwards, my good days were 2 or 3 per month, from that, I started to notice certain things. I could do things that I could not do before, the headaches were getting less, the actual strength in the body was changing, my emotional strength started to change, I started to see what was draining me and I started to think differently towards these.

I began to spend more time reading, which was so wonderful, finally I could focus on words again.

My body pain started to dissipate a bit, then I started not to think about these issues that were consuming me before. I was able to walk and for the first time I did 2 kilometers by myself without stopping. That was great and the dogs loved it.

One of the things I had enjoyed before the illness was to take my Staffishire Bullterrier Fred, on a walk every morning before the kids woke up.

So it was one of my goals after the illness, to be able to do this again.

Which I did, slowly at first, also the elements were an issue, the cold affected me a lot, I felt so sensitive that the wind felt like it was hurting. When I would touch my forearm muscles they felt bruised. My throat was swollen red and sore every day.

I would go to the doctors only a few times because they said they could do nothing, they would take bloods with no results. I stopped going, it was futile. I changed doctors several times in the hope that I would get some sort of help, but it was ridiculous, I remember one of the doctors, said oh maybe you don't have CFS (I just wanted to burst out crying, I had had CFS for 8 years then, as if I would not know the symptoms of this horrible pain by now) I am able to forgive the doctor now. There was another doctor who said I don't think you have CFS you probably have gallbladder problems so he sent me off for investigations which came back negative.

These symptoms were beginning to simply, not be there, every single day like they were for years.

It was exciting, it was hopeful and I started to build up strength everyday.

Now, I have strength and I can throw a punch if I wanted to and not fall down in a heap for 3 days straight. I have body strength, I can do sit ups, I can run, which is something I could not do before, any cardio exercise would have me collapsed for days. I ran up the hill twice last week. Just because I could. I burst out laughing by myself. It felt great.

Dancing, and even drinking vodka with orange, staying up till 3am in the morning, I did that for my sisters hens night. I felt ecstatic to do this, it was a wonderful memory. It was also not the only time I did this, I have done it several times since. Something I could only dream of in these past 9 years.

Thank you Ashok!, thank you for your dedication and help.

Chapter 12

SLEEP

It is a well known fact that the body repairs itself when it sleeps. Therefore the chronic fatigue sufferer's need for sleep is vital. Now some of you may be thinking, but all we ever do is sleep, we do not have the energy to do anything else. Nevertheless, would you agree that we also stress about the fact that we are resting while we have so much to do? Is that thought not stressful? Refer to Energy Chapter for more information about 'energy drainers'.

We may not be making time, to clear, or change, the things that we need to, allowing our body to heal and enjoy better sleep. We need to stop and think about the things we need to repair in order to have a good night sleep. We must make this one of our main priorities because sleep is the body's optimal "repair time."

The "Health Goal Affirmation" exercise is a very important tool for putting into perspective what we need to work on now. As well as focusing on:

- Our health and achieving the progress of healing.
- Next we need to look at our gut function. Raw Diet.

- Then the stressful activities to release the symptoms of stress.
- The detox plan.
- Followed by looking at things we need to change to improve our immune system.
- Attending to our pain.
- Reviewing the possible changes that can be implemented after reading this book.

As we prioritize our time, especially when we begin to feel strong, we can work through these suggestions. It is not an easy 1,2,3 step solution, but it is definitely a great guide to produce strong results in the healing process.

Once these have been worked on, you may find that your sleep pattern starts changing. Remember to complete the breathing exercises before bed time and as you wake up, they are very important. They will allow a pattern of centering and calming the central nervous system.

HERBAL PRODUCTS

Talk to your Naturopath about a combination of herbs or single herbal tonics to address your lack or quality of sleep. There is a range of middle and strong herbal tonics available.

I found an extremely small dose of Passion fruit Flower herbal tonic combined with the liquid herb Valerium works well for me. I keep to a small dose because I do not want to over use it and therefore reduce the effect. I use it like a homeopathic solution taking 3 to 5 drops under the tongue straight, undiluted. This usually sends me back to sleep pretty much straight away. Remember that the effects of herbs vary from person to person and the effects of the additional medication you may be on, need to be taken into account.

You may like to discuss with your Naturopath using Nux Vormica 30c, which is a homeopathic solution generally used for liver issues. But if you have a tendency to wakeup around 2am or 3am, these time relates to the liver meridian and Nux Vormica could be of use.

HINTS AND TIPS FOR IMPROVING SLEEP PATTERNS

- No heavy exercise before going to bed.
- Meditation prior to sleeping.
- Complete breathing exercises.
- No coffee, this for some reason has a distinctive effect on the liver and if you must have a coffee you need to have one only and very early in the morning, same as black tea or coke/ Pepsi/cola other stimulant drinks.
- Double check you are not taking vitamins that are not recommended before bed, e.g. vitamin B (which can have a stimulating effect)
- Sugar in any form before bed.
- The following exercise is a Kinesiology correction to balance the right and left brain function/energy.

EXERCISE: BALANCE RIGHT AND LEFT BRAIN

- Place your left hand over your right hand and your left foot over your right foot. Take a few breaths and hold the pose for 5 minutes then relax.
- There is also a sleeping/snoring ring you can purchase at some chemist/pharmacies which has a little ball at the end of

the ring. It is an open ring, in the shape of a U, this helps by putting pressure on the meridian that runs on the inside of the little finger. Some people find it very useful.

- Stop snoring aromatherapy product can be found at the chemist or health food stores.
- Using Lavender essential oil (please remember that some lavender oils have been combined with chemicals and this can be highly reactive for some people. This reaction is similar to some perfumes which contain chemicals that give chronic fatigue syndrome sufferers an allergic reaction. Always purchase lavender essential oil from either a health food store or a naturopath and check the labels. Use essential oils only. Be careful.
- Place a few drops of essential oil in a spray bottle with water and spray the room.
- Use a journal. Write down anything that is playing on your mind, put it down on paper. Often this allows stress to be released, as you see it on paper you see different solution, like a mathematical calculation. You can find ways to deal with the stressful issue and therefore it helps you to de-stress. Even if you do not find a solution while you a writing the issue, it is on paper and you can come back to it later. Essentially it is out of your head.
- I have found the sleep and brain function of stress release is one of the last symptoms to leave the body once you start to heal. This illness leaves you feeling very raw, in reference to releasing stress quickly.

EXERCISE: IF YOU ARE STRESSED OUT ABOUT THE DAY'S EVENTS

Cross your hands left over right hand and legs also left over right leg for 5 to 10 minutes.

Take slow breaths in, pause then breathe out, several times to regulate your energy.

Visualise the infinity sign (the number eight placed in a horizontal position) trace it with your mind's eye.

Take note, when your energy starts to come down and you begin to feel more relaxed. Release the arms and the legs and breathe.

You may feel the body tingling. That is a good indication that the energy has changed.

EXERCISE: LIGHT ON THE PINEAL GLAND

During the day make sure you get the 10 minutes in the morning and 10 minutes in the afternoon of sunlight on your forehead. This helps to regulate the pineal gland in charge of sleeping patterns. (This is great for anyone working shift work).

If you are unable to get natural light, use a torch or even visualise the sun on your forehead. This is a very important exercise and much research has been done on the pineal gland and its effects on the body.

EXERCISE: MUSCLE CONTRACTIONS

This exercise is simple. You need to relax and contract your muscles one group at a time. Let's start with your feet and calves.

Squeeze these muscles hard and then let them go and then allow them to completely relax. If they are very tight you may like to repeat this exercise several times on a certain area.

Then slowly work your way through your body. Move to the upper legs, repeat the relaxing/contracting exercise. Continue to work your way through your body, the buttocks, the stomach, the arms, the chest, etc. By the time you get up to the head you can squeeze your eyes and then relax, frown and then relax, make faces and then relax. It is quite interesting to note where you were holding much of your stress.

SOUP FOR DINNER

Having a heavy meal, especially something that will be hard for the body to digest can definitely affect your ability to sleep.

Whilst on the raw food diet I noticed a significant improvement with my sleep pattern. When I eat meat, sauces or heavy food at night my body can react to heavier foods with burning leg symptoms, hot flushes, restless legs, achy joints, creaking and cracking of the joints, my stomach feels hot and swollen and my face and hands feel puffy on waking.

These symptoms do not appear when I eat meat occasionally. However, if I eat meat for several days or weeks, then it takes me several weeks to get rid of the above symptoms. Not to mention the symptoms of a sore throat and bad breath. This not only happens with meat, fish, chicken but also sugar or sugar drinks just before bedtime. It does not happen when I eat fruit or drink freshly squeezed fruit juices and I am on a strict raw food diet.

EXERCISE: HUMMING

Using the sound Om or Amen and letting it vibrate through your body will release any stuck energy in your body.

So you breath in and as you breath out you say Om or Amen slowly and let the sound vibrate through your body.

Meditation before bed is great. Allowing your thoughts to settle and concentrate on your breath.

Sleeping well, engages much of the bodies mechanisms. Lack of sleep should not be taken lightly, as it is a major aspect of healing. It is very useful to use a good enzyme complex after meals especially at night, where I have personally found a significant action in symptom reduction.

The general sleeping pattern that is experienced by a CFS sufferer is, collapse as soon as you go to bed, then wake up mid night with an overactive brain then 1 or 2 hours before you have to wake up if your lucky you fall asleep again. The pattern is interrupted and very unsettling. I use valarium and passion flower liquid herbs a few drops during this time of broken sleep and it generally helps me to fall back to sleep. As I mentioned in other chapters once the gut starts to repair the sleep pattern starts to improve and your central nervous system seems to settle down and you get a full night sleep. And you wake up feeling good.

Chapter 13

DEPRESSION

Depression in CFS people, I feel could be described as, a de-pressed state, compressed, squashed, contained, not flowing, stagnant, restricted, low in energy. Not to be confused with a mental health disorder from birth or a psychological fixed chemically imbalanced seen as clinical depression. Even though a developed depression derived from years of suffering CFS may progress into depression.

There is considerable feelings of shame attached to what is described as depression and the connection of western medicine practitioners to prescribe anti-depressant medication for CFS diagnosed patients.

It's given to patients not only to help them with the symptoms of depression, but, to help them with the over active brain, anxiety and the pain as I understand it.

Many people have expressed that they found themselves depressed after developing CFS because of a few reasons, one they are not believed, two the doctor may say they can not help them leading them to a feeling of helplessness, three they do not know where to turn, to heal, four the illness goes on for many many years, five the therapies and products do not give them an instant result and six because the illness affects them in all aspect of their lives.

Today, there are many people with a variety of views on anti-depressant medication. When I express my view on this subject it is not given as a recommendation but solely as my own personal view. I find it could be useful for other patients not a top priority for CFS sufferers. Anti-depressants, the medication; the composition; the effects, including the side effects; the "stigma" and its affect on the psyche to me are controversial for a CFS sufferer. I feel the CFS body is very sensitive and an allergic reaction could manifest to some antidepressants, which sometimes can take months after stopping the medication for the brain and body to settle down again.

People believe in the benefits and what you believe is the only thing that is pertinent and must be important to you. If you use it and it works for you, go for it.

What options do you have? Some suggest products or techniques, using St Johns Wort herbs, tincture or herbal tea or even homeopathic remedies as well as minerals and many other natural remedies.

ZINK, is probably one of the most under estimated supplements that we have on the shelf. When I had post natal depression, it took me a week of taking Zinc liquid, again not in tablet form, it is not effective, to regain my strength, and overcome the symptoms of post natal depression. I could not believe how simple it was! I recommend you talk to your naturopath about the different options for depression while experiencing CFS.

Your naturopath can view your body and retrieve information for example:

Why do my nails have ridges?

Your fingernails' health can tell a great deal about your internal health. These abnormalities of the nails are often the result of nutritional deficiencies or other underlying conditions. Here are some of the nutritional deficiencies and what they do:

Hangnails: Lack of protein, folic acid, and Vitamin C
Brittleness and dryness: Vitamin A and calcium
Horizontal, vertical ridges, and fragility: B vitamins
Excessive dryness, rounded and very curved nail ends, darkened nails: B12
"Spoon" shaped nails and/or vertical ridges: Iron deficiency
White spots: Zinc deficiency
Splitting nails: Lack of hydrochloric acid

Also a horizontal dip can indicate a stress you may have experience, could be emotional or physical, like a heart attack, or even heart break some response to set your fight and flight mechanisms flying.

I personally have had an interesting manifestation of a stressful event I experienced after being heart broken, my nails showed a dip in the nail two weeks or so after the event.

I have put together some exercises following, to help with the now sensitive body and central nervous system you may now be experiencing with Chronic Fatigue Syndrome.

PROTECTION

The CFS sufferer would benefit by understanding not only where they are losing energy, the colander effect, but how to protect themselves.

The body has not only become sensitive to chemicals, foods, environmental factors but also to emotional attacks.

When a person has high energy levels, they can ward off, quite easily, those criticisms or digs that your friends or ex-friends, family, acquaintances, boss, etc, might have given you, but now that your world is so raw, the nervous system is just not behaving like it used to.

Some ideas of protection are as follows:

When you have been criticised for example and your body has gone into the reflex, fight or flight mechanism, remember to take a deep breath. This changes the shock state and allows flow again, the breath is very powerful and will get you moving again. It can allow you to calm down in the fight reflex and it can help you flee calmly.

As the breath is taken in deeply, it performs a very distinct reaction in the travels of the red blood cells in the blood system, as opposed to sedate shallow breathing, I was just reading a physicist explain.

PROTECTION WITH COLOUR

View a bright, sparkling white light around you, before the event or even during the event. If you know that usually you experience a negative reaction or confrontation with a certain person, using the white light can be a pro-active exercise in protecting your weak body and psyche.

EXERCISE: AVOIDANCE

Avoiding certain situations.

Don't think yourself weak for organising to avoid a certain conflict or person or food for that matter, you are actually being strong for doing it. It takes strength and courage to plan and look after yourself especially when you don't have the energy to think about what you are going to wear let alone thinking of negative circumstances.

So for example, you may have a family member that seems to engage in fighting with you on a regular basis.

First acknowledge. Once you acknowledge that this is actually happening, then you can make a decision or take action, for example say to yourself how important is it for me to be heard, be right, be acknowledged, be respected, be noted, be thanked by THAT person (this could also be a circumstance), what is my priority, is it to heal? If so, you acknowledge to yourself, that this will now be your priority and if this person you can see makes you feel tired, weak and exhausted after having minimal conversations, then take the action and delete time spent with this person.

Then watch your energy grow, day by day. It will be amazing.

EXERCISE: EFT, EMOTIONAL FREEDOM TECHNIQUE

This is a great technique which I recommend. I have used this on myself as well as with my own clients. Best to search on YouTube and spend some time understanding exactly how this works. (confidence and self worth meditation with EFT).

I find it very useful when you are confronted with a stressful situation for example, taking some time even if its locking yourself in the bathroom for a few minutes and tap away that stressful comment or feeling that was stirred up.

For example: Even though Kate has said I always forget to pick up the mail and called me annoying, I still love and approve of myself. Then tap on the meridian points that are shown on the film clips when you have searched the technique on YouTube.

EXERCISE: USING MANTRAS

Mantras are used to raise the vibration of the body in a positive way. It uses repetition and vibration, the humming is used to unblock any stuck energy in the body.

Thoughts do have an impact on the body.

According to quantum physicists on a subatomic level, everything is a form of energy, or patterns or wave of light and sound frequencies.

That is, everything in the universe vibrates. The earth is made up of specific frequencies, including our body, and even the mantras.

Einstein has also correlated matter and energy, and that energy interacts with matter. Therefore, since a mantra or thought is energy, and matter is related to energy, therefore any change in mantras or thoughts could produce corresponding changes in the matter.

Like prayers and mantra healing, use this principle when they heal and improve the condition of our body.

Japanese scientist Dr Emoto researched that positive words have high vibrations, and they positively affect the water crystallization process producing intricate shaped water crystals. Whereas, negative words have low vibrations and they created chaotic and deformed patterns of water crystals.

However, mantras are the thought power houses and source of high vibrations. Mantra healing definitely affects us and the environment in a much greater manner, bringing about order at the subatomic level. This process can also help heal our body parts and organs.

Cleve Backster is another scientist who observed that the plants generated polygraph results that were identified with happiness on good treatment with positive thoughts, while the results were opposite with negative emotions. After many studies on the impact of thoughts on a number of living things, scientists concluded that even living cells and bacteria are subject to be affected by our thoughts and the power of mantras.

So the use of a POSITIVE THOUGHT or a POSITIVE WORD can have and do have a reaction on the body.

An example of a mantra that I use is:

Thank you for my healing.

I am healed.

This is repeated many many thousands of times.

EXERCISE: USING VISUALISATION

Visualising yourself soft and transparent when being attacked helps you to become flexible, letting it pass through you. By not confronting the attack, letting the negative energy just go through you, it passes without affecting you. This takes a bit of practice but a good tool.

EXERCISE: THE CEASAR MILLAN TECHNIQUE

I have coined this technique as the Ceasar Millan Technique. I thought it was funny. Be assertive, own your space and treat the attacking dog, or person for this exercise, with a grounded assertiveness. Practice saying "No, do not hurt me, no, down" or "ch." I actually said that once to my husband, (ex-husband now) who was yelling at me at the time and looked like a ferocious dog. I said "CH stop that!"

It confused him long enough to stop yelling.

EXERCISE: THE GREAT ESCAPE

Walk away from a situation that is causing you pain. Emotional pain is and can be physical pain and it vibrates sometimes for days in your body. Move away from the "fire" as they say.

If the person who is attacking you or confronting you face to face, i.e.. you are facing each other and your bodies are too. Move your body to one side and let that negative energy past, do not take it on with your body being directly front on to the other person.

EXERCISE: DISTRACTION TECHNIQUE

This technique is using a distraction action. This is used again when there is a negative or confronting situation that you feel is stressing you out. Use an action that is totally out of place to distract the situation.

An example would be to start hoping on one foot, start singing, smile, pull a face, do a clicking noise with your mouth, pull your hair, rub your ears, etc, get creative. This action has to be strong enough to get your mind out of the stress situation at hand.

EXERCISE: MUSIC TECHNIQUE

Everyone has their own taste in music, but it is undeniable that it has a very strong effect on the body and has been well documented and studied. It has abilities to lift the mood and depression.

Dr Emoto has done some great work with documenting the effects of certain songs on the crystallization of water, I recommend you view his work, it is quite inspiring.

When I met Dr Emoto, in Sydney, a lovely man very humble, I thanked him for the work he did and he was so gracious, his energy was amazing. His wife ran around organising things around him she seemed very devoted. Both very dedicated to the work.

I remember that day it was a seminar he did in Sydney on a Wednesday night and I had to travel 1 and 1/2 hours to see him, they had to change venues because he had such a large turnout. The whole presentation was translated into English as he spoke. People in the the audience were able to ask him questions after the seminar, the energy in that auditorium was amazing, he has now passed away so I feel very privileged to have thanked him in person.

In reference to music, just as an example of a song that I found inspiring, Kelly Clarkson, Makes you stronger (what does not kill you) I am sure you have some wonderful music you can relate to, that does have an uplifting affect on your psyche.

EXERCISE: LAUGHTER TECHNIQUE

Exercising laughter on a regular basis has been connected to effects on the heart, lungs, gut area and muscles. There is some research findings that laughter has an affect on diabetes and eczema, heart disease and asthma as well as depression. It has been shown to increase immune function and help fight infections. There are laughter therapy sessions sometimes conducted by yoga teachers, who incorporate the laughter technique with other techniques such as clapping and chanting.

Laughter can increase levels of natural killer cells (lymphocytes), boost levels of natural pain killer, improve anti-inflammatory activity and reduce levels of the stress hormone, cortisol. Some studies have also shown a good laugh increases levels of the "cuddle hormone" oxytocin and melatonin, as well as the brain chemicals serotonin and dopamine, both of these chemicals are what antidepressant medication address.

EXERCISE: CUDDLE TECHNIQUE

This technique, not only oxytocin and melatonin levels can increase but also have a lasting effect on the central nervous system. The pituitary gland secretes Oxytocin hormones. This gland is part of the endocrine system which is certainly affected in chronic fatigue syndrome sufferers.

You can do this by asking someone else to hug you or you can hug yourself, holding tightly with your arms wrapped around you.

It is very effective when you have anxiety.

EXERCISE:ANTI-ANXIETY TECHNIQUE

Using a scarf long enough to wrap around your arms and back, wrap it around yourself and hold it tight for a few minutes until the anxiety decreases.

When you start to get anxious again hold your arms around your body and visualize someone hugging you.

Do the breathing exercise of taking a breath in slowly 1,2, hold for 1,2 then breath out for a count of 1,2.

Also hugging your pets is effective.

MOULD AND DEPRESSION

Dr Mercola, Dr Cheney and Dr Constantini have important information on mould and its overlooked effect on depression. I found Dr Mercola has some wonderful information on these effects and he quotes some laboratories that can do some testing in the USA for moulds. He talks extensively on mycotoxins which are toxins produced by mould or fungi.

Dr Hulda Clark and her work on the Zapper machine and her detoxes is also very important reading in reference to CFS symptoms and fungi, bacteria and parasites.

Some alternative depression products suggestions to look into are the following: Kava, L-truptophan, Saffron, St John's Wort, blue-green algae, omega 3 fatty acid, Goji, Homeopathic remedies, Lavender, Lion's mane mushroom, Motherwort, Valerian, SAME and many other products.

Chapter 14

HOME AND YOUR ENVIRONMENT

As a matter of priority, it may be good to check what plants are growing around your home (where you live, work and sleep) Have you noticed for example that roses growing in the yard, do not flourish and they get black spot or aphids? In your environment do the weeds: chickweed, milk thistle and/or oak trees thrive? These plants do well over ley lines and some plants are overly affected by black spot or aphids when planted over ley lines.

GEOPATHIC STRESS

Studies done in Germany regarding geopathic stress lines (also known as ley lines or energy lines or underground water lines or veins) are showing a correlation between the frequency of ley lines and patients with Chronic Fatigue Syndrome. As well as Fibromyalgia and other chronic illnesses like Cancer.

This subject is important for anyone with a long term illness that is persistent many studies have been done especially in Germany, view www.natures-energies.com.

I personally took this information quite seriously and even though it took me many years to make the decision to move away from a particular bedroom where I had two ley lines crossing, my health has had a significant improvement. I had two separate practitioners test the house for ley lines and they both came up with the same information, regarding where my bedroom was located. I feel that once your strength starts to recuperate, then your body can manifest significant health improvement.

You can find some companies addressing this phenomenon, such as this one called geoclense in Australia view www. orgoneffectsaustralia.com.

Types of Geopathic Stress dealt with by the Geoclense products are the following:

Negative Effects Eliminated by the Geoclense Device
Negative Effects Eliminated by charged metal plates
Negative Effects Eliminated by EMF filters
Negative Effects Eliminated by Holographic Imaging Technology
Negative Effects Eliminated by organite based devices

Earth Magnetic Grid Lines

Earth magnetic grid lines or ley lines are known as standing waves of electromagnetic energy, emanating from the ground and high into the atmosphere. Some of the different types include Hartman, Curry, Benker, Cathie and 400M grid lines, which vary from around 300 mm wide as with the Hartman grid, to 6 meters wide as with the 400 meters grid lines.

Electromagnetic Radiation

Electromagnetic radiation is a strong source of dangerous positive ion produced by our electrical systems and appliances. Some appliances, such as washing machines, fridges and multi point power boards create very strong and large electromagnetic fields. Electromagnetic radiation (EMR) is measured in milligauss using a device known as a gauss meter. In countries where the governments are concerned with the wellbeing of the people and the effect of EMR on their health, milligauss readings from electrical systems have guidelines to ensure that people are not exposed to readings of 4 milligauss maximum. It is known that EMR readings of above 4 milligauss have been known to cause childhood leukemia and cancer in adults. There is also scientific evidence that high exposure to EMR with women can cause a dramatic drop in melatonin levels and a link to breast cancer.

Underground Flowing Water, Sewerage and Grey Water

Underground flowing water, water veins and water flowing through pipes under our living spaces are another source of dangerous positive ions. Water veins resonate at around 13 hertz, and create a noxious energy field to around 1500 mm above the ground. Cats love to sit above water veins because the water veins are around 2 degrees warmer than the ground either side of them. Sewer and grey water create a noxious energy field due to the resonant cavity effect of the water and waste traveling along within the pipes.

Seismic Fault Lines

Fault lines create positive ion fields above ground level in varying widths and directions. Often they contain the memories and energies of emotional trauma associated with historic massacres. Geomancers and spirit workers with knowledge on how to clear the emotional imprinting within the fault lines, area are easily able to clear the noxious energies from fault lines.

WI FI Fields and Beams

Wireless communications of varying types such as mobile phones, wireless Internet, local wireless modems and routers, and even baby monitors all create strong positive ion beams which link from device to device, and/or to transmission towers. Should any of these beams penetrate a person they can create a feeling of nausea, mental instability and a greatly compromised immune system.

Paranormal Interferences

Imprints from the event of the death of a person, and subsequent Spirit Lines create dangerous positive ion fields. After someone has passed away, the actual place of transition after the body has been removed creates what is known as a death imprint. A subsequent spirit line may emanate in the north south, or east west directions. Should the person who has passed become stuck on the earth plane as an ethereal being, then the spirit of the person is bound to the imprint and spirit line. The danger is when someone spends time over such energy fields, then the spirit has an opportunity to infect the persons various chakras as an attachment. The infected person can show traits of personality and ailments similar to the spirit when they were alive. Here again, a trained geomancer or spirit worker is able to clear the noxious energy imprints and help the ethereal being spirit to a higher plane.

Mould and Fungus

Mould and Fungal growth both create strong dangerous positive ion fields. We often find mould growing under floor boards or under old carpet that has been exposed to spillages or other sources of moisture. Poorly ventilated bathrooms and laundries are particularly prone to mould and fungus. The resonance created by mould and fungus can totally overcome the energies of a given space, and again can be a greater danger than EMR from electrical appliances and wiring should you be sensitive to it. The symptoms generally are respiratory complaints and mental instability.

New Noxious Energies of the 21 Century

HAARP Beams

These beams we believe are a by product of the military over the horizon radar systems, which are scattered around the world. Their purpose is to be able to see incoming missiles before they come over the horizon during times of conflict. Haarp beams are also possibly an aural research platform, so we are told. However the operation of HAARP creates an intense radio frequency beam of around 300 mm in diameter which impacts the earth every 5 meters square to north, coming in at an angle of around 45 degrees to the ground. These beams are extremely dangerous to our health as we see so many people with systemic health issues in the body which correspond to exactly where these beams have impacted upon their bodies while they are sleeping. We believe that the HAARP Beams have only been around since roughly the year 2000.

Personal Beams

Personal Beams, not to be mistaken with personal lines, which are of no real consequence, tend to be abundant wherever you find people sleeping or where they sit for prolonged periods of time. They come vertically up out of the ground, and in the case of sleeping arrangements, run across the neck. Or when sitting, either directly through the chest, or along the length of a couch. They then stop 3 to 5 meters beyond the person being targeted. The personal beams are similar to the HAARP beams in size of around 300 mm in diameter; however we believe them to be similar to a microwave beam. This is how some researchers who have the ability to see energies perceive it.

please view www.orgoneffectsaustralia.com/Geoclense.

I purchased a gauss Master Meter to measure EMF, so as to arrange all electrical devices at a safe distance and to check the EMF from what I used daily.

Its best to turn off all electrical power points in your bedroom and make sure you do not sleep near the house meter box or a high tension wire tower near by in the street.

The following information below is from www.rolfgordon.co.uk, I was quite fascinated by this concept and from my personal experience I recommend, that you may like to have your bedroom and house checked by a Feng Shui practitioner who does dowsing.

"Geopathic Stress is the only common factor in most serious and long term illnesses and psychological conditions.

It was proved to the satisfaction of the medical profession over 80 years ago and in millions of cases ever since, that Geopathic Stress is very detrimental to human health.

Thousands of medical doctors and therapists now confirm that any Geopathic Stress (GS) must be cleared before any treatment can be 100% successful.

The most common indications of GS are :- Resistance to medical treatment, a feeling of being run-down and exhausted, nervousness, depression, loss of appetite, pallor and not wanting to go to bed and when in bed: insomnia, restless sleep, feeling cold, cramps, tingling in arms and legs, sleep walking, grinding of teeth and nightmares. When waking in the morning often feeling fatigued, with a muzzy head and backache. Children are often bed wetting and babies continuously crying.

GS does not cause an illness, but lowers your immune system, so you have less chance of fighting any illness. GS also prevents your body properly absorbing vitamins, minerals, trace elements etc. from your food (and supplements) and often making you allergic to food, drinks and environmental pollution."

CLEANING PRODUCTS

My experience with bleach has been one of when I have accidentally touched and smelled bleach I got sick, had to lie down, felt weak and my head was spinning. Recently on the market is a product called bleach but the reactions to white cotton does not coincide with the usual bleach. It makes the white cotton have a reddish mark instead. What can this reaction be? Again are we being sold bleach or a different cheaper alternative under the brand of bleach which we have not been made aware?

There are many ways to clean the house without chemicals; there are also many of us that like the house to smell clean. But it's the smell and the chemicals that cause such a negative impact on our health.

CFS and chemicals do not mix well and I feel you need to learn to delete chemicals from your household cleaning products. I do relate to some people who have been brought up using chemicals to clean and if the house does not smell like disinfectant it's not clean.

Here are some ideas to replace them with:

Bicarbonate Soda (Bi carb)
Dishwashing liquid
Dry: scouring the pots (or use bi carb and vinegar and leave, then wipe clean it's so easy.
cleaning metal
floor cleaner
bench disinfectant then polish with a cloth

(Remember: Bi carb is a great Alkalinizer and germs do not like alkaline environments)

Vinegar
Neutralizes smells clean garbage bin
Toilet cleaner
Pet odours
When you bring fruit and vegies home wash with one table spoon of vinegar in the tub full of water.

Both Bicarb and Vinegar makes a froth leave overnight on cook top and oven then clean in the morning it lifts dirt and grime.

Salt, sterilize the chopping board with heaps of salt and let it dry.

There are great books on Vinegar uses. You can look up Bicarb uses with www.mckenziesfoods.com.au

There are some companies which are doing some great work regarding keeping the environmental and sensitivity issues at the top of their aim. There are many great products available including Herbon, view www.Herbon.com.au or another example www.envirocareearth.com.au.

PERFUME

Under this section I discuss the sensitivities that CFS sufferers now face on a regular basis.

There has been a significant connection between people with CFS and reactions to perfume, deodorant, and air fresheners. Whether it's a particular chemical added to fragrances in the last say 20 years or simply that CFS sufferers are overly sensitive to them. If you search Dr Joseph Mercola's and look up the archives of when he spoke to a researcher who advises that under the word Perfume there are about 300 chemicals that the government has decided, were not necessary to be disclosed. This is very interesting and informative.

A useful tip here is that if you have had a reaction to something you inhaled, like bleach, paint or heavy disinfectant, using an antihistamine or anti-allergy tablet from the chemist seems to help.

Everybody is different and will be affected by all sorts of different perfumes, some will have reactions and some will not.

My view and something that's worked well with me is using rose water and/ or orange blossom water, which is used for cooking and cosmetics etc instead of using perfume or commercial deodorizers. You can buy rose water in the supermarket in the cake making section, make sure there are no additives.

I use rose water and or orange blossom water in a spray bottle for:

Breath freshener
To clean your skin and as a toner
Underarm deodorant
Clothes deodorant
Ambient deodorizer
Foot deodorant
Perfume

As a cleaner with a little bicarb (dilute with water in spray bottle) and clean the fridge, the kitchen benches, the bathroom tiles, floors, basin, shower.

I also use lavender oil. This needs to be essential oil and I prefer to buy it at a Natural Therapies clinics. They usually carry the good stuff, if this essential oil is cut with cheap oil, you may be in a bit of trouble. Some people have bad reactions to the carrier oil or the chemicals that they have put into it.

I use lavender oil diluted in water in spray bottles the same way as the rose water. Sometimes I find it useful to have alcohol (small amount) in the spray bottle to clean the toilet and basins, it makes a good disinfectant. For disinfectant use, you may like to use teatree oil or eucalyptus oil.

Buying some lavender flowers and placing them in water on the stove for about 10 minutes on low heat to extract the essential oil, makes good and practical lavender water for use around the house.

You can use this technique with roses; after you enjoyed watching the flowers don't discard the old roses take the petals and make rose water the same way as the lavender you can do the same with other flowers like jasmine, orange blossom, or herbs like peppermint, spearmint, lemon balm, rosemary and other herbs in the garden.

MOULD AND FUNGUS

I have researched information on this subject regarding, the effects these may have on a person with CFS or any person who has a compromised immune system. By the way you may come across doctors who think that the immune system of the person with CFS is not compromised. I do not agree. So I look at my health issues as if my immune system is totally wonky. I feel strongly that my immune system does not function correctly. The amount of viruses and reactions that I have had, do not show me, that my immune system is strong at all.

There is some evidence that some moulds and fungus can affect and compromise the immune system. If they are present all the time, it is hard to know what is the stimulating variable, what is affecting the body (mould for example) being the stress activator. So sometimes physically moving home or taking a very aggressive and proactive approach to ridding your environment of black mould, fungus overgrowth etc. is when you will notice that it was, in fact, having an effect on your symptoms of CFS.

You can have an allergy test where the skin is pricked and the mould is placed directly on the skin to see if a reaction forms. The only question I have with this form of testing is that it is not long term and sometimes the symptoms only appear after a long time exposure to these moulds. You need to evaluate and investigate this form of stress for yourself.

Just a thought, use plenty of vinegar to kill mould in the bathroom or window sills. Keep the bathroom well ventilated, and if you are in the bedroom for long periods, change to another part of the house and make sure you ventilate and clean the room regularly. Keeping free of dust, build up of dirt and other cumulative moulds and fungus bacteria are very important.

Attention must be kept on anything that can be considered as a low lying infection or stimuli to the immune system. In my case the long term exposure to gold, (gold molar) had a profound affect to my energy levels.

THYROID DYSFUNCTION

Chronic fatigue and thyroid dysfunction, is there a correlation between these two?

Pesticides Damage Thyroid

25 February 2010: Your thyroid gland plays an important role in regulating your metabolism and energy use. There is growing evidence linking pesticides to thyroid problems. This study examined 16,500 women living in Iowa and North Carolina who were married

to men seeking certification to use restricted pesticides. They found that twelve and a half per cent of the women had thyroid disease with seven per cent having underactive thyroids (hypothyroidism) and two per cent having overactive thyroids (hyperthyroidism). In the general population the rate of diagnosed thyroid disease ranges from one to eight per cent. The study found that organochlorine pesticide use was associated with a 1.2 times greater risk of hypothyroidism. Exposure to fungus killers benomyl and maneb/mancozeb doubled or tripled the chances of hypothyroidism respectively. Maneb/mancozeb also doubled the women's risk of hyperthyroidism. The herbicide paraquat almost doubled the likelihood of hypothyroidism. Yet another example of how your environment can impact your health.

Source: American Journal of Epidemiology

MORE ON MOULDS AND FUNGUS

I have been using Zeolite powder to deal with mould and fungus as well. I did a little experiment where I had an onion which had a cut through it and green mould was growing on it. The smell that was coming from this onion was quite strong. I placed the onion in a bowl and poured zeolite powder on the onion and left it for 2 days, the smell had gone and the colour on the mould had changed. I left it for a further 2 weeks on my bench and the onion did not smell. The mould did not disappear but the smell was gone.

I now use Zeolite powder to clean my benches, my sink in particular and I use it every day to wash my hands, it takes out any smell and its specific purpose is to remove chemical build up.

If I want to remove any odour or smell from something I use Zeolite powder quite effectively.

I use www.nikitanaturals.com.au to purchase my zeolite powder. You may like to subscribe to McKenzie's 160 Bi-carb Soda tips and uses booklet, its free, to get your copy "Like" them on Facebook.

Chapter 15

PRODUCTS AND THERAPIES

CFS patients have unusual reactions and sensitivities and therefore benefits from products, services and therapies will vary.

There are many product and services that have provided a great deal of relief in symptoms for their consumer or clients as well as many products and therapies that have been built up, maybe for marketing purposes to portray amazing results but have had not delivered results for the CFS sufferer.

The cluster of symptoms that make up Chronic Fatigue Syndrome can be viewed individually or can be viewed in groups for example by body systems that they derive from, vascular or endocrine system and then from that perspective, I would choose products to target that particular area or system.

However we know that Chronic Fatigue Syndrome is not a simple illness and that it affects people uniquely. There are many variations to the cluster of symptoms from client to client. I feel it depends where each individual carries his or her weakness.

For example if you have a client with a predisposition for neck pain due to a car accident, it is likely that the neck will become a key feature in the pain experienced. If its lower back then the pain can be more intense in that area instead.

It is very easy to be discouraged by the continuos and costly exercise of trying new products or services and I have heard many people comment "I am not trying anything else, nothing works" (purely out of frustration).

It is such an individual decision and thats why its called personal choice. I have also noted that the attitude that you bring into an interaction with a product or service has a significance in the outcome. As doctors refer to it, the placebo effect.

Having a background in Health Science and an interest in nutrition, herbal medicine and homeopathy, as well as running a naturopathic clinic for 12 years, my choices in products and services have been towards the natural type. I also use pharmaceutical products and feel there is a place for everything we have available. As I have often heard, "you don't go to your naturopath when you have a broken leg," you go to the hospital. There is a place for everything.

In my own personal experience with the trial of many products especially when I was very ill and unable to get out of bed, I had come across many products that did nothing at all to change the symptoms, not one bit, even though the manufacturers claims where so impressive. It was disheartening and annoying and of course costly so I know exactly how some people feel in this regard.

In my opinion when the body is overloaded and not functioning well as in toxic symptoms, many products don't help because the body is overwhelmed. All the way through your illness and most importantly when you first get sick with CFS is **to reduce your stress dramatically and detox your body.**

Learn quickly to stop the body from using up your precious energy in stress related actions and reactions. So it has the energy to concentrate on healing in order of priority.

Allow the body to heal by keeping it very quiet and still, pay attention to the breath and pumping of the lymphatic fluid by using deep breathing with gentle contraction and stretching of muscles.

The pain experience in the muscles is thought to be that of lactic acid build up. Similar to what athletes develop after running a marathon. The elimination organs need a great deal of attention. Such as bowels, if you suffer from constipation, do not let that be, do everything possible to release the bowel movements regularly. Keeping it stagnant will only allow the body to reabsorb the toxins.

Water intake is used for flushing so, drink often and use preferably slightly alkaline water. A few leaves of parsley in your cup of tea helps the kidneys to flush. Take note of all the different cleanses under the detox chapter. Pay attention to the gut, eat raw and green juicing to heal the gut. This will work on the inflammation of the body and the pain will start to get better. Its not a matter of putting a few juices in your daily routine, its about 90 to 98% raw food intake. This is strict.

PRODUCTS FOR GUT FUNCTION

One of the common problems with CFS patients is gut function, and malabsorbtion of the gut wall, due to candida, IBS, malfunctioning digestion, food allergies and stress. Here is a list of products in relation to gut function.

Spirulina: It has over 120 naturally occurring nutrients with more iron, B-12, carotenoids, trace minerals, enzymes, EFA's, antioxidants and phytonutrients.

Acidophilus and Bifidus: There are a few on the market and recently they brought out one with 8 strands. There is also some that are available for storage in the pantry instead of the fridge. Cannot comment on the difference, I have tried both.

Peppermint Tea as well as ginger: Useful for nausea.

Sugar: Say good bye to it for a minimum of 6 weeks better 3 months.

Enzymes: Life Style Enzymes is just an example of a company who produce enzymes, one of their new products does not use sulphites (which some people are allergic to) something to look out for. There are many digestive enzymes on the market.

Essential fatty acids: Eg: fish oil, flaxseed oil, hemp seeds, walnuts, black currant seed oil, evening primrose oil. The balance of Omega 3 and 6 is very important. Your naturopath can advice here.

Probiotics: Probiotics help the immune system by competing with unwanted organisms for nutrition and oxygen and therefore altering the acidity levels in the gut. They also help with pathogens in the gut. (An over growth of parasites seems a common problem with CFS patients)

Colonics: Hydro Colonic Irrigation, helps with parasite overgrowth, cleans the bowel and hydrate the body.

CleanseU: as a parasite control and bowel cleanser. There are other products like this one which your naturopath can combine for you.

Natural enzymes: Paw Paw (papaya), pineapple. Use every week.

Natural anti viral, anti bacterial food: Coconut (eat plenty of this amazing food) raw.

Alkaline water: Will assist many bodily functions.

THERAPIES FOR PAIN

Remedial massage, lymphatic drainage, very slow and very gentle strokes will help to move the system around, you do not want any of these toxins to pool in any area of your body. So even though it may be uncomfortable or you feel sick the next day. I would highly recommend a gentle massage followed by a day of rest and heaps of water and green tea for the next few days.

You can use Yoga in this same way to move and contract and relax certain muscles which in turn work on certain meridians which in turn feed certain organs of the body, so yoga is invaluable as a form of wellness and giving your organs a helping hand.

Swimming is wonderful as it is gentle on the joints and even just floating and moving slowly in the water helps the lymphatic system to move. Not keen on the chlorinated public pools I find I react to the chlorine especially when I am feeling sensitive. Salt pools could be an alternative and the ocean and fresh water rivers would be ideal.

Osteopathy and physiotherapy, very hands on modalities which can address pain very specifically. Once the central nervous system is relaxed by you paying attention to everything possible that you can do to calm down the system with breath, meditation, cognitive therapy, mindfullness meditation amygdala retraining program, etc, then you can use Osteopathy and physiotherapy effectively but not when the pain levels are still quite high.

I feel that if you just tackle the pain with hands on techniques like osteopathy and physiotherapy without also addressing the calming down of the central nervous system, it can be more painful. Thats only my view and experience. Also make sure that you are well hydrated before your treatment sessions.

Meditation: Many studies have been done on meditation and its affect to lower blood pressure, and reduce anxiety. For CFS sufferers it is something that needs to be done every day on your own. I would recommend to attend a meditation group at least twice a week.

So to recap, the useful products and services that I personally have used with success are, colonics, Gupta amygdala retraining programme, herbal mix called "CleanseU" made in Australia, gingko herbal liquid, valerium and passion flower liquid herb, homeopathic nux vormica 30c, rescue remedy (bach flower remedy), and eating raw food, juicing morning and night and salad at lunch, including smoothies and raw soups. Water, bicarb soda, zeolite powder, lemon and vinegar, for energy boosts CoQ10 by Metagenics.

MY STORY

At the beginning of the illness I had no idea what was happening to my body. The symptoms, plus the variety of things that were going wrong with me, it was all too much. It was hard to make sense of these symptoms and even harder to find professional care.

My family did not understand how I felt and I interpreted that to mean that they did not care. So I started pretending that it was all going to go away soon and I was not going to care for myself either. I would pretend there was nothing wrong. I worked, I slept (more like collapsed) I could hardly speak, let alone focus on anything. I am not sure how I took care of the kids, but I did, and we all survived.

My illness started a few months before my 40th birthday, within a few months I experienced the following:

It was exam time, the last year of my Diploma of Health Science and Remedial Massage Therapy.

At exam time I learned my grandmother had cancer with a poor prognosis. She raised me from birth till the age of 10 years old so we were very close, I travelled to South America and spent time with her, three weeks later she passed. The second major tragedy was the death of my beautiful sister in law Melanie. An off duty police woman at the time and was killed in a car accident, she was only 20 years old.

We put our house on the market which sold in a matter of weeks. We had to pack up the family home and move quickly to my in laws.

I had the responsibility of mother, student and home maker whilst managing our naturopathic business and starting my own remedial massage business while my children where 6 and 9.

My father underwent an emergency quadruple bypass three days before that Christmas.

Plus I had a complicated root canal therapy that year.

In addition to these highly stressful situations in my life, which took place within a 16 month period, my blood tests results indicated evidence of Epstein Barr Virus. Prior to this, at the beginning of my CFS symptoms I had no signs of a virus. I did not feel unwell, I had plenty of energy and I was bright enough cognitively speaking to undertake study with my Diploma. So it was quite startling to have those results showing that I had previously experienced the Epstein Barr Virus.

Roughly 4 months before developing the CFS symptoms, I did have a very bizarre and scary experience. I was in Sydney for the weekend attending a workshop on Kinesiology in Neuro Organisational Technique with Bernard Carson a wonderful and very talented Kinesiologist. I had arrived the day before and stayed with my parents in Sydney to save on traveling time. My sister suggested going out for a few drinks to a local club. That night two men approached our table and chatted with my sister. I remember going to the bathroom while they were there and when I came back they were gone. My sister and I were drinking, but because I had such a huge weekend planned with studying, I only drank one glass of red wine and sipped my sister's strawberry daiquiri. Plus my sister and I shared dinner at my parent's home that night.

During the night at the club, I started feeling very strange. I felt I had to get out of the club as I was very uncomfortable and just felt weird. I asked my sister if she minded if one of her girlfriends drove her home because I just wanted to go to bed straightaway. I then made my way to the club car park.

I walked past a security guard kept walking and as I was approaching my car I felt uneasy, as if someone was looking at me and I turned around and there were the two men who were talking to my sister and her friends earlier. They made me feel very uncomfortable and I began to get frightened and very wary that these guys were walking too close to me and there was not enough time to make it to the car and lock the door. So I had to think quickly, I turned around so fast walking briskly towards the security guard, that when I did this, the men had to move away from each other as I had passed in between them.

I pretended to look in my bag for my keys and chatted to the security guard, while these men kept looking back at me as they continued their walk across the car park towards the street, they did not even get into a car at the car park.

I ran towards my car and locked the doors and drove off when all was clear and made it home in about 5 minutes. That night I vomited 13 times, I was so terribly unwell. I still attended the course feeling very foggy brained the next day.

I suspect that these guys may have put something in my drink that night. As I understand the date drug commonly used, gives the victims blackouts and foggy brain as well as vomiting or nausea. Thank goodness I have a strong constitution and was only 5 minutes away from where I was staying.

The common drugs used for what is called date rape drugs, are GHB (gamma hydroxybutyric acid), ketamine and rohypnol. Other street names, Liquid ecstasy, Grievous Bodily Harm, Easy Lay and Gamma 10, Mexican Valium, La Rocha, roche, Roopies.

If the drug used that night was rohypnol, which tests positive when I muscle test the name (a kinesiology technique) then the symptoms experienced makes a great deal of sense. However there was no proof because I did not think of going to the doctors to get tested at the time.

Rohypnol is a brand name for flunitrazepam (a benzodiazepine), a very potent tranquilizer similar in nature to valium (diazepam), but many times stronger. The drug produces a sedative effect, amnesia, muscle relaxation, and a slowing of psychomotor responses. Sedation occurs 20-30 minutes after administration and lasts for several hours.

Well, since that experience my symptoms of CFS started getting more prominent and more visible, four months later I went to see Dr Gow, who tested me for Epstein Barr Virus. He thought I had glandular fever. I also went to seek a second opinion with a Doctor in Bowral and he confirmed it was Chronic Fatigue Syndrome. So, since then,

I have been trying to repair my health and do a great deal of research on the subject.

During the next 7 years, I tried many different treatments before coming up with the 4 Techniques that helped me to change my life. They are:

1. COLONICS
2. DETOX PLAN
3. HERBS (Cleanse-U Plus Gingko)
4. AMYGDALA RETRAINING

For the first 12 months, I took colonics fortnightly and once a month for the next 12 months. Now it's a few times per year.

The detox plan was Dr Ian Rafter's detox plan, which is simple, so simple, that I almost did not do the plan at all. I knew the effects of this detox plan on people with Autism, Dyslexia, Attention Deficit Disorder and Hyperactivity and was very familiar with the studies done in reference to these disorders.

The plan is: no wheat, no dairy, no sugar, no alcohol, and no coffee.

For a period of 6 weeks minimum, though 8 weeks is even better.

To actually get an exact period of 6 consecutive weeks with no wheat, no dairy and no sugar, was challenging to say the least it took me 3 months to achieve it. It takes quite a bit of effort getting your head around these requirements. And there is a lot to learn about the foods that contain wheat, dairy and sugar, a lot to read and attention paying on packaging.

You also need a good understanding of what is dairy (no butter, no cream, no sour cream etc) Sugar appears in almost everything in the supermarket, so going to the fruit and vegie shop is it. Don't even bother going to a supermarket. If you have to shop there, please read the "Sensitivities chapter" section of my book. I would recommend the raw diet which I did on a 90 to 98 percentage raw for 2 months straight and then reduced the raw to incorporate slowly other foods. But I find keeping to at least a 60 to 90 percent raw diet will keep the inflammation at bay and you certainly notice this regarding body pain.

For the first time my fog brain had lifted and I could read again. I wanted to read and I was retaining the information. I can understand the non desire to pick up a book, in fact, it almost repels you, the mere thought of it.

Then came the wonderful Naturopath Eli Shamon, in Parramatta, Sydney, he has put together a herbal tonic to help with quite a few aspects of the detoxing process, the tonic is called "Cleanse U," and I have been taking this for the last 9 years, and still take it, with great success. Some people feel it is hard to take mainly because it can cause a lot of bowel movements, but if those bowels do not move how is the detox going to happen? Another great little gem is the Gingko herb for memory. Bitter as anything at first, but knowing its great effects, you soon get used to it.

Occasionally if I have problem sleeping, I take the herb Valerian and Passion flower. I take it straight, a few drops on the tongue is all it takes for me. I also find it helpful if I have a stress response to something or someone or even an allergy reaction.

For energy I take CoQ10, the brand by Metagenics, and find it works fast and effectively. To keep my thyroid in balance I take Thyrobalance and for adrenal exhaustion Adaptan from Metagenics as well. Also liquid herbal mixes for the thyroid or the kidneys, what ever needs attention at the time.

The herbal teas I take are: Peppermint (for nausea and because it tastes nice) St John's Wort (for mild depression and immune support) and Gingko (for memory) I find it works well to combine these teas and take them daily.

The next major step towards recovery I had was with Dr Ashok Gupta's Amygdala Retraining Program, I bought the DVD and attended a few of his seminars on the web. I found this program helped me tremendously by curving and understanding the importance of stress management and its affect on the Chronic Fatigue Syndrome symptoms.

Once I mastered the technique, my body began to start repairing and healing. The days in bed became less and my resistance to viruses was getting a lot better. This process is slow and an attentive mind is necessary I also documented my feeling and my progress to see if there were changes.

Which, there were, but everything happens so slowly that it is understandable how some people may overlook it.

Then I started some serious Stress investigations. I had my house checked by two separate practitioners in the dowsing field and both detected I was sleeping over a ley line or water veins, the area where the bed is placed is over 2 ley lines crossing actually. I have moved to another area of the house.

One last bit of information I'd like to share is that for years I had a feeling that my gold molar was weakening me. It was put in place, after having root canal therapy, the year I started to get sick. I thought maybe there was an old infection underneath the molar. I knew that something was wrong, I just did not know what it was exactly.

I had asked my dentist to remove this molar many times, during the 8 years I attended his clinic. He insisted it had nothing to do with my CFS and it would not be a good idea and the two were simply not related.

I finally went to a different dentist, who said exactly the same thing, except this time I did not listen. I insisted I wanted this molar taken out. It was finally removed and I spent some serious time doing detox with Zeolite Powder. I knew it was important to purge my body of the toxins.

In powder form, I used it as a mouthwash, toothpaste, hand wash, foot wash, underarm, bathed in it, soaked my feet in it.

The results were significant. My energy levels have been increasing dramatically, and I had noticed my resistance to viruses has also increased. Instead of being in bed for days and even weeks I was recovering within 1 to 2 days. I was getting so exited with my results. Yet I know that only people who have recovered from CFS could understand my happiness.

I remember telling my dentist how good I was feeling, and him looking back at me with such a puzzled look on his face, I am sure he thought I was over reacting. Even when I spoke to my current general practitioner, he also looked at me with the, sure lady whatever look, when I told him of my new surge in energy.

Another significant change that had occurred was that I had stopped working with my husband at the clinic. The stress of working closely with a questionable partner is not something I would recommend. The importance of reducing stress was becoming more apparent. The quest to reduced stress was having an effect on many aspects of my life, including the decision to start paying attention to and seeking therapy on my body's structural issues. I had 2 slipped discs in my neck where one area was encroaching on my nerve. Working on the realignment and healing with a physiotherapist and acupuncturist both in Bowral NSW, had made a great deal of difference to my neck and even my vision.

My experience in experimenting with a raw food diet has been very successful and with exceptional results. My skin has changed, my strength has increased, quick recovery from illness such as a flu or bug have improved. Plus I even felt like running up hill which I can do now regularly. I have gone for bush walks up to a 14 kilometer hike up and down mountains. My recovery was so surprising it is very encouraging. I am very excited about continuing all these treatments and being able to share my findings with you.

Be aware that following the raw food diet is not that easy. I have deviated several times already, and every time my body lets me know. On reflection, it is so visible when I get bogged down with foods that is not high in energy my energy levels suffer.

When a CFS patient is feeling good, you need to sit up and take note. This is not a common occurrence – but thankfully since I have made significant yet achievable changes to my lifestyle, my diet and personal habits, I am continually feeling so much better.

Well, that's my story so far. It may seem strange for some, but others who are experiencing CFS, I know you will relate to at least some aspects of my journey.

CONCLUSION

Sometimes out of something hurtful or perceived a bad situation or comment can come a brilliant insight or break through and that's where I found the final piece of my recovery puzzle.

A very close person to me said, 'I wish you had cancer and died because putting up with you being sick all the time is unbearable'. After getting over the shocking words coming from someone you love so much, I began to think about the fact that I actually knew people who recovered from Cancer and they healed themselves, so I thought may be I could heal myself from CFS too. From this, emerged my final boost of energy and recovery. It came from these wonderful people those amazing survivors.

I find that in chronic fatigue sufferers the hyped up central nervous system is so wound up that it affects the endocrine system, the hormones, the sleeping patterns, the brain, the muscles as well as the heart in a way that is disruptive.

Calming the central nervous system is the KEY, achieving this using will power, meditation and breathing techniques and of course I found the Amygdala retraining program was and still is invaluable.

Detoxing and actually understanding what detoxifying your body means and how to put this into action daily.

NOTE: Find what GIVES YOU the most stressful response in your body. This is particularly critical because we are all different.

Where you are loosing energy or where energy is being taken up unnecessarily, for example, constant exposure to certain chemicals, or amalgams or gold crowns or any other dental product that your body is reacting to. It could be something like sleeping over geopathic zones or ley lines or may be a chronic stressful relationship, or work environment, cleaning products, inhaling fumes etc. I experienced another significant and gradual burst of energy when my ex-husband decided to stop talking to me he left after a year and a half, I was noticing that my energy levels were getting better, I was so excited in getting my energy back that the pending divorce did not register much.

There are several very important facts but I think the base is deleting sugar, wheat, dairy, coffee/black tea, alcohol for at least 3 months. This will have an affect re setting the immune system, like a reset button on the computer. You don't necessarily need to be on this strict diet for ever just long enough to destroy the candida overload and repair the gut function. Detoxing the system and resting is just as important, 2 to 3 months on a raw food diet while taking a very large green juice every single morning.

How did you feel about the sensitivities chapter, have the concepts there helped? Has it clarified or intrigued you into viewing some positive aspects of Chronic Fatigue Syndrome?

The four main techniques I discuss, which are, colonics, detox diet, herbs and the Gupta amygdala retraining is the basis of the process of releasing symptoms of Chronic Fatigue Syndrome.

As you start to release yourself from these negative impacting exposures you start to understand the exercises that assist the calming of your central nervous system, with the techniques discussed you will develop adjustments that accumulate into positive tangible and distinctive symptom changes. You will notice your symptoms start leaving your everyday life. The wonderful thing is, that you experience healing gradually and unmistakably.

NOTES

SUPPORT GROUPS

Chronic Fatigue Syndrome Society SA Inc.www.sacfs.asn.au
www.fmcfsme.com
www.me-cfs.org.au
Western Sydney: facebook, ME/CFSsupportforSWsydney
Action for ME (UK) www.afme.org.uk
Alison Hunter Memorial Foundation, Sydney .www.ahmf.org
Co-Cure ME/CFS and Fibromyalgia Information www.co-cure.org

BIBLIOGRAPHY

Pesticide Chemistry and Toxicology By Dileep K. Singh
Complete Yoga By Stella Weller
The western guide to Feng Shui Terah by Kathryn Collins
Colon Health by Dr Normn W. Walkers
You can heal your life by Louise L. Hay
Pollution Solutions by Harald W. Tietze www.wise-mens-web.com
It's so Natural by Alan Hayes
Power vs Force The hidden determinants of Human behaviour by David R. Hawkins MD, PhD
Love the life you live (Workbook) A ten step life coaching process by Anne Hartley

Wildly Happy and Wise by Maggie Wilde
The vortex by Esther and Jerry Hicks
Geopathic Stress by Rolf Gordon www.rolfgordon.co.uk
The body is the barometer of the soul by Annette Noontil
Anatomy of the Spirit by Caroline Myss
The secret language of your body by Inna Segal
Your year for change by Bronnie Ware
Health for all by Harald W. Tietze www.wise-mens-web.com (wonderful naturopath)
Bicarbonate of soda by Diane Sutherland, Jon Sutherland, Liz Keevill and Kevin Eyres
Change your thinking by Sarah Edelman Phd
Ley Lines and Earth Energies by David Cowan and Chris Arnold
Light Emerging by Barbara Ann Brennan
Crystal Colour and chakra healing by Sue and Simon Lilly
Hands of Light by Barbara Ann Brennan
The Synchronicity key by David Wilcock
The power to heal by Robert Pellegrino-Estrich
Encyclopedia of healing juices by John Heinerman
Raw Logic by L R Murray Fruit and Vegetable juice therapy

THERAPIES

COLONICS
www.naturaltherapypages.com.au
www.nutrition4life.ca
www.livestrong.com
NATUROPATHY
www.karunahealthcare.com.au
www.australiannaturaltherapistsassociation.com.au

ACUPUNCTURE

www.christopherbooth.com.au

www.acupuncture.org.au

PSYCHOLOGY

www.psychology.org.au

REMEDIAL MASSAGE

Australian Traditional Medicine Society www.atms.com.au

OSTEOPATHY

www.osteopathy.org.au

HEALING

www.inner-truth.net/healing/chakras/crownchakra

YOGA

contact Tafe or Adult Education College in your area

THAI CHI

contact Tafe or Adult Education College in your area

AMYGDALA RETRAINING PROGRAM

DR Gupta in the UK

www.guptaprogramme.com

DOCTOR

Dr Ian Rafter, Australia

Index

Printed in the United States
By Bookmasters